Her FATHER'S HANDS

a journey of health and healing

LYNELL CAVNER

Cover photo: Analise Cavner

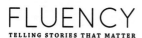

Produced with the assistance of Fluency Organization, Inc.
Design by Inkwell Creative

To all who are on their colorful tour,
searching for their purpose.

I hope you find inspiration through my
words and know that whatever your
situation, "This too shall pass."

table of contents

acknowledgments

To Alexia Monroe, my Bowenwork Instructor. Thank you for teaching me so well on the mechanics of Bowen/Bowenwork, as well as for your encouragement to actually put it into practice fully.

To my husband, Pete, and my daughter, Analise. Thank you for being ever so patient with my long hours and my attention to so many others throughout the years. Your steadfast support and love for me means more than you will ever know.

To Dad, William Louis Schafer. Thank you for instilling in me common sense, patience, and perseverance. All three have served me well on many levels of my life.

To my late Mom, Jean Ann Schafer. Thank you for having been a strong role model in my life and for teaching me many principles of faith-based living and how to live with confidence in my abilities. And thank you for being a guiding mom, even from your deathbed.

To my staff, Denise, Debbie, Suzanne, Ann, and Natasha. Thank you for putting up with all my "pineapple" ways. To Suzanne, specifically, thank you for helping with all the typing to ensure this book becomes a reality.

To Robb Martin. Thank you for being such an inspiration of hope! You are one of the most peaceful, joyful people I know. In my mind you are the epitome of "we are made in God's image"....healing from the inside out even after so many years! Thank you for allowing me to be part of your healing process and inspiring me to write this book.

And most importantly, to God. Thank you for never giving up on me with all my wandering. Thank you for blessing me in my dreams and in my life...allowing me to be a vessel of healing for others by you.

about the author

LYNELL CAVNER IS THE founder and owner of Lynell & Company, a Body and Nerve Restoration Center in Prescott, Arizona. She earned her bachelor's degree in Holistic Nutrition and is a Master Certified Bowenwork practitioner and Associate Instructor. A farmgirl at heart, Lynell is a native of Michigan and has been living and working in the Southwest since 2002 where she established her business in Prescott, Arizona.

When she's not at work, you can find Lynell out on the trail running with her dog, swimming in her pool, or undertaking another gardening project around the house. She has a natural love for the outdoors, physical fitness, and staying busy. Lynell is a fighter for her clients, an advocate for the body's natural ability to heal itself, a believer in food as medicine, and someone who leads by example in the protocols she recommends to her clients.

Lynell and her husband, Pete, and their daughter, Analise, live in the beautiful community of Prescott.

www.LynellnCompany.com

1

my father's hands

MY FATHER'S HANDS may have looked like any other farmer's hands, but there was something extraordinary about them. Well-worn from a lifetime of working outside, they carried scars that told stories about how he'd hurt himself trying to mend a fence or fix something on the tractor. When he was milking his cows (four at a time), he made sure they felt loved and comfortable, washing and massaging their coats while they did their job. I imagine our cows were the only ones in our county who might recognize a Tanya Tucker tune, since Dad often played country music in the background while they were being milked. Some people may have laughed at the personal attention he gave to them, but his 65 cows produced more milk than any of our neighbors with more than twice that number.

Dad also had an intuitive way of monitoring health with a touch. With those same rough hands he could lightly touch a distressed animal to diagnose what was wrong, and he also had the uncanny ability to know when we weren't feeling well. Throughout my childhood, I watched Dad curl his weathered palm around the back of one of my sisters' or brothers' necks, and within a few seconds he told Mom what was wrong. He could sense ailments from strep throat to a belly ache with surprising accuracy. Mom would then take us to the doctor in town for a professional opinion, only to learn more often than not, that Dad had indeed been right.

When I was little and suffering from an ear infection one day, Dad lit a brown cigar, cupped his hand lightly around my throbbing ear, and gently blew the grey smoke into it. He smiled and told me to be sure and plug the other ear with my finger so the smoke "wouldn't come out the other side." That made me giggle, and I suddenly realized my ear didn't hurt anymore. Mom looked at Dad with a knowing smile, and I understood something like magic had just taken place in our living room.

My family sometimes teased Dad that he should have been a doctor, but he would always shrug off this unwanted attention. We knew our father would rather work with animals, not humans. Still, his gift remained as undeniable as it was mysterious. My dad's lifelong interests were always somehow related to his hands. He was a sharpshooter in the military when he was a young adult, cradling his rifle with a steady grip that enabled him to focus on his targets. Dad said that once he calmed his nerves and focused, he could feel in his hands how the gun was going to respond. Those same youthful hands being trained for battle also wrote Mom the sweetest love letters at night before he went to bed. In his letters, he wrote about the day's events and assured Mom that he couldn't wait to come home soon and ask her to marry him.

When Dad bought the first 140 acres of our farm in his twenties, he worked a blue-collar job to pay for his dream. He was a tired and busy man and later added neighboring acreage as it became available until he had expanded our family farm to 365 acres. For fun, Dad pitched for a local baseball team. Many nights the seven of us and Mom filled the wooden stands at the baseball field alongside our neighbors and others in our small community to watch Dad throw knuckleballs and sliders, striking out batter after batter. Dad was as comfortable holding a hammer as he was a baseball, and he could fix or build anything. These same hands that molded so much of my childhood would also play an unexpected role in my own future at a crucial time in my thirties when I needed direction.

I never saw Dad rush. "Hurry, but don't rush," was his motto. His walk was more like a saunter, but he accomplished so much every day because he never stopped moving.

He always said the cows on our farm were better watchdogs than our dogs. Dad named many of his cows and called them by name when it was time to go inside the milk house in the evening. They responded whenever he called them in from the pasture as sure as if he were calling to one of my siblings or me. He rarely raised his voice—not to an animal and not to us at home—but my father absolutely ruled the barnyard like a king with a scepter. He kept his pitchfork nearby for the regular occasion when one of the bulls acted up, as the testosterone-driven males were prone to do. Dad would raise the pitchfork above his head and slam the metal end on the dusty ground, which startled them and made them stop misbehaving immediately.

When it was the season for cutting hay on the tractor, we would often come upon tiny fawns carefully hidden by their mothers in the tall stalks. Occasionally, a frightened fawn wouldn't run away in time to avoid getting injured as the tractor made passes through a field. My father would stop the engine and step off the tractor, wrap the terrified animal in a towel, and bring it up to the house for me to tend to its wounds. He taught me what to do to treat the injury and calm the animal so it would not be afraid.

I learned early on through this experience that feeling safe is essential to healing. If an animal felt safe and not threatened in any way, their body would relax, and they might eventually even sleep in my arms. The hours I sat silently tending to wounded fawns passed quickly for me. It would often be a week or more before they were strong enough for my father to return them to their anxious mothers awaiting their babies in the woods.

I loved animals and spent many quiet hours holding everything I could hold in my arms, from puppies who wouldn't nurse to sickly calves who needed to be bottle-fed. My family also raised several litters of cocker spaniels. I remember when one of our dogs had puppies and she decided on a whim to move her babies one night from a box on the porch and hide them in the dark green stalks of the corn field. When Dad came in from milking the cows about 11:00 that evening, we were all sound asleep in bed. He always made the rounds outside to check everything after he finished milking, which is how he discovered the puppies were gone and immediately began looking for them. When my father finally heard their cries as he reached the endless rows of corn in our field, he turned and promptly sauntered directly back to the house to wake us up. Within minutes, we had boots on our feet and flashlights in our hands, headed outside into the night.

By the time we carried the last armful of crying puppies back to the house, an hour or two had passed. I had a knowing feeling as we packed the puppies back into the box that the mother was likely going to move them again. We didn't know why she didn't want her babies on the porch, but it was clear to me that she was agitated despite all our gentle soothing. After everyone else went to bed, I snuck back outside and stuffed all ten of those guys one-by-one in a box under my bed for the night. I shared a room with Jillayne, one of my four sisters, and she sleepily muttered something about hearing puppies barking outside under our window. I just smiled and crossed my fingers, saying nothing, since we both knew our mom had an obsession with cleanliness and didn't like animals being in the house. The puppies eventually slept through the rest of the night undiscovered, but by morning it was no use with their loud barks and yelps, and I got in trouble.

At least once a week our family would visit my dad's mom, who lived about five miles away from our farm. She and her brother were from the Netherlands and immigrated to America before the Germans invaded. The two of them recounted their own adventure on a ship going across the Atlantic. They were sponsored by an American organization that connected Europeans like my grandmother and her brother with working class families. These families were welcoming enough, but in truth they were often looking for free help on the farm, not necessarily adopted family members to take care of.

The work was long and difficult, and my grandmother gradually earned a hardness about her as a result. She met and married my grandfather in America. He was German, which made Dad was half German and half Dutch and made me a mix of the two, plus Irish on my mom's side. I didn't know my grandfather because he had a heart attack and died while driving his tractor when I was in first grade. What I do remember was their Gran Torino we called The Pig for some reason. It was quite the car—green as could be and fast, although my grandmother never learned to drive. When my grandfather was alive, there was no need to learn because he drove her anywhere she wanted to go. She was a true tulip queen from the Netherlands and could plant anything and make it grow. It didn't matter what it was, she could grow it. Best of all, she was an excellent baker, and every Sunday after church she served us homemade fry cakes (which were like cake donuts). We would dip them in what she told us was coffee, although what she served the children was actually just a steaming cup of milk with lots of sugar and a dash of coffee. It was delicious.

We spent most of our time with my mom's parents because they lived closer. I often walked the two miles or so to their house by myself to spend time with them. My Irish grandparents made an interesting pair because he was slender as a reed, and Grandma was this large, round woman with a lap so warm and inviting that you just wanted to crawl up, settle in, and take a nap. Because of her weight, she had trouble moving when she was older. I recall the many visits Mom and I would make to help "walk Grandma." We made a few laps around the kitchen table just to keep her active. Afterward, I massaged her legs that were very swollen with accumulated fluid. She seemed very old to me for her age.

Grandma would often pass out glass jars for us to catch fireflies, a wonderful tradition I remember of my summers in Michigan. She assigned each of my siblings and me a specific number to catch so that we would stay busy. That way she could visit in peace with my parents. We had to catch as many fireflies as we were years old, a clever strategy for also teaching us to count at the same time!

When we caught the appropriate number, we poked holes in the metal tops of the jars using a screwdriver so the creatures could breathe. Grandma assured us before we left for home that she would use the glowing insects as nightlights to lead her safely to the bathroom in the middle of the night. I'm not sure that was true, but it's what she told us. She routinely called each of us the next day to thank us for our hard work. Grandma let the fireflies go, of course, emptying the jars the next morning so we could repeat the whole routine the following week.

Grandpa was a consummate farmer with an Irish temperament that made him both fun and fiery. He was a lot like my oldest brother Daryl—you either loved him immediately, or you couldn't tolerate his over-the-top energy. All my uncles were hellions, according to my mom, and she had often stepped in the middle to break up fights between her dad and her brothers.

Daryl and Grandpa lived wild and large. As the oldest boy, Daryl pushed us all to be daring and take chances. He couldn't understand why anyone hesitated in life when he would just go for it. Whenever I cut loose, I was more like the two of them—rambling Irish roses without a care in the world. Grandpa lived to a spry 95 years of age and remained active throughout his long years. Before he died, I had an unexpected experience that prepared me for his death. So when that day came, I was at peace. I had often imagined my fun-loving brother would grow up to be much like his grandfather in his old age, but it wasn't meant to be. Nothing in the world could have prepared me for the shock of losing my brother.

You didn't mess around in our household, as Daryl learned repeatedly throughout his teenage years. At home, my parents were very clear about what was expected of us. They matter-of-factly informed us of the rules, along with what would happen if we chose to ignore or disobey those rules. Mom and Dad never argued in front of us, and God help you if you crossed one of them, because one was swift to support the other. Dad would not put up with Daryl sassing my mom. They had each other's backs at all times. We were generally well-behaved, but it was Daryl who would get us all in some sort of trouble most of the time. And it is Daryl who is woven into so many of my childhood memories.

Up in the haymow (a loft in the barn where we stored hay) there was a hole in the wood floor where we pushed shovels full of hay to the hungry and badly-behaved bull that lived alone in exile in the corral directly below. One day Daryl decided to string a rope from a rafter and dared all of us to swing over the hole. We had to hold on to the rope for dear life because if someone didn't make it safely to the other side, they'd be down there with the bull! And he did not want company.

Daryl also managed to convince us on more than one occasion to grab hold of the electric fence after assuring us he had turned it off. The fence was designed to keep a 1000-pound cow away, so naturally when we touched the live wire it zinged us! He thought that was so funny, until Mom came flying out of the front door of the house determined to get him. I don't know how we survived so many of Daryl's bright ideas. I also lost count of how many times I was almost electrocuted in my childhood!

I half-jokingly say that my hypersensitivity to electric jolts from Daryl's tricks may have even helped my career. I have a quiet suspicion that I might not be far off from the truth, as I am an associate instructor and practitioner in Bowen therapy and also the CEO and founder of Lynell & Company, a Body and Nerve Restoration Center in Arizona. I've always been unusually perceptive with people and animals, both on an emotional and physical level, and my sensitivity to their feelings and experiences rarely fails me. And sometimes it even surprises me. My work with clients is very intuitive as a rule. I will sometimes understand something about a client's pain based on intuition that later turns out to be right. It's reminiscent of my dad's gift, and I don't claim to understand it, but it happens.

There is a positive and negative side with any gift we receive, of course. The day I touched what felt like hot razor blades in the neck of my best friend, Karen, I instantly sensed it was an aggressive form of cancer. She had been acting strange lately, struggling more than usual to find a word and even saying the walls in my house looked like they were arcing when we were hanging pictures together one day. "My arm feels like it has too much coffee in it," she remarked one day. "It's all jittery." We didn't know a brain tumor was growing inside her head. A gift can be a blessing and a curse all at the same time when an instinct turns out to be tragically accurate.

Dad very rarely watched our television on the farm because he didn't have time. Whenever he had a few spare minutes in the evenings, Dad enjoyed watching the *Nightly News* with Tom Brokaw. Being so far out in the country, our TV produced an unreliable picture anyway with lines crisscrossing the screen. When the picture became unwatchable, one of us would have to trudge outside to adjust the large antenna on the roof. One night when I walked through the living room, passing about three feet away from the TV set, the picture suddenly became crystal clear.

"Whoa!" Dad said, holding up his hand. "Back up…"

I did, wondering what he meant.

"Stay right there," he ordered, not taking his eye off the TV screen. "That's perfect."

No one had to brave the weather and adjust the antenna that night, and Dad got to finish his program! It's a weird party trick, but sometimes if I'm near a staticky radio or TV, the signal will suddenly come in clear. One day in the clinic a set of speakers in one of the treatment rooms was picking up a lot of electricity in the dry Arizona air. All I had to do was wave my hand around the face of the speaker and it would emit a "vroom...vroom" sound that my staff all agreed was kind of cool and creepy at the same time.

My siblings and I are all very different, but we all loved each other and had to learn to work together as a unit on the farm. In high school, if one of us wanted to go on a date, we had to work it out with our other siblings. Dating taught me how to work with family members to get what I wanted. You either finished your chores in time to leave the house to meet your date, or you got one of them to cover for you. That was the deal. If they didn't want you to go on your date, they could make it so.

I was very sociable in high school and loved to go out. What is the worst Mom or Dad could say if I asked to see my friends? If they said no, I couldn't go out with a boy, I just invited him over to our house instead. Problem solved. More than once, my siblings hinted that I got away with more as the youngest girl because our parents were tired out by the time I came along. But I got to do more because I asked, that's all. I was always negotiating, and Dad eventually said I could go out on Friday or Saturday on a weekend—but not both. He always seemed to know what I was up to, and I often thought that was because I was so much like him. Dad had many friends and loved to laugh and tell stories. People enjoyed talking with him. I also have a lot of Mom in me. She ran a tight ship, and so do I. Her teacher-like authority comes out in my personality at work and at home.

Growing up on a farm, I witnessed nature's cycles of birth, illness, and death up close with both humans and animals alike. My parents never sheltered us from experiencing the difficult parts of life. Nothing was ever hidden from us. They didn't teach us to avoid discomfort, and we learned at an early age to enjoy life while also learning to deal with inevitable hardship, heartache, and pain. One of my extended family members who grew up in the city struggled so much when my mom's mother died. We were both teens, and I remember being amazed that he couldn't get it together enough to go to her funeral. I thought that was unusual then, but I've learned that many people resist death as a normal part of life. Whenever one of my animals died on our farm, I accepted it. If you had to put an injured animal down, you just did it. It's not that you become hard-hearted living on a farm, but you learn perspective, and you come to a valuable understanding of how life operates. As Mom often said under her breath after every crisis, "This too shall pass." I would have plenty of opportunities in the future to see that she was right.

I also grew up with a natural sense about prioritizing health, and that was true for our family, our animals, and the crops we grew. We all worked hard outside for many hours every day, day after day. Mom would kick us out of the house and say, "If you're not throwing up or having diarrhea, get outside." In her book, being in the fresh air and sunshine would heal most anything that was wrong with you. My siblings and I learned never to say "I'm bored" on a farm because that would lead to being assigned another chore. "There's a rake in the garage," Mom was always ready to suggest whenever we had time on our hands.

The benefits of hard work and outdoor exercise were ingrained in me from the time I was a child. We spent hours painting fences, raking the yard, or feeding cows. We ran narrow trails in the forest in our free time, spent whole afternoons on our tire swing, and scoured the woods for wild berries in season so Mom could make one her famous pies. All of this emphasis on being active and outdoors would come into play much later with the clients in my practice, but I did not know that at the time. I was just a kid playing hide and seek with my family, tucking ourselves behind the cows so no one could find us.

My mother also did all the cooking at home, not to mention a lot of the tractor driving in the fields. The closest village was three miles away. It had a teeny grocery store where Mom could call the butcher and request certain cuts she wanted. We grew most of our own food and traded eggs or milk for other items. Mom had a big area in the backyard reserved for our family garden, and every spring and fall we helped plant a variety of vegetables that would soon end up on our plates for dinner. Squash, watermelons, carrots, turnips, and green beans (my favorite, whether on the vine or bushel beans) grew well in the rich Midwest soil. My father planted sweet corn for us alongside row after row of regular corn to feed his cows.

My sister Jeanette and I were allergic to dry hay and

couldn't be outside during hay baling season. Mom was out driving the tractor working with the rest of the family, so we did the cooking. I was 10 and Jeanette was 15, and we rolled up our sleeves and prepared hearty batches of food for the family and field hands who often joined us—a total of about 19 people.

Mom had certain beliefs about the qualities of specific foods. For example, if we ate red meat at a meal, we had to pair it with broccoli or some other dark green vegetable for better digestion. It's no surprise that it's much more natural to me as an adult to turn first to food for healing, not a pill or a bottle. I am well-versed in the natural healing properties of specific foods because I was raised with that understanding. I didn't consider it unusual, and I thought everyone knew what I knew about the healing potential of food! But as I began working in the health industry, I realized how many people have absolutely no reference point for a natural, organic approach to food and its healing potential.

My parents modeled and taught us about the importance of mental health also, even though they certainly didn't realize that's what they were doing at the time. Dad's advice about life and his gentle guidance came naturally in opportune moments—while we sat with him on the tractor, or when we were busy painting or pulling ears of corn. On a farm, there is very little time for sitting around, shooting the breeze. From sun-up to sundown, every member of the family was busy pulling their weight. Mom also chose her moments to convey the most important lessons while we were distracted by everyday life. She could whip up a complete meal faster than anyone I've ever known. It was like magic—and that's when we did a lot of our talking in the kitchen working alongside her.

Unfortunately, I also saw my full-blooded Irish mom steep herself in worry throughout my childhood. She liked to be in control of everything and was also a neat freak, determined not to have a dirty home! I can't recall all the nights we went to bed while she was cleaning the counters and dusting shelves in the living room. We were on the lower end of middle class and did not have a lot of money, but she made sure our home was beautiful, inside and out. She liked to say that just because you are poor doesn't mean you should be dirty! "Cleanliness is next to godliness" was another one of her favorites, and like the teacher she was for most of her life, she controlled all of us the same way she took charge of her classroom. The problem was that we were not as compliant as her students. Mom and I would go toe-to-toe often because I did not think her standards were realistic, considering we lived on a farm where dirt is part of everyday life. Plus, she worried too much about the people and things she could not control. She didn't quite know what to do with me and had a hard time controlling me most of all, because I challenged her out of her OCD quite nearly every day!

If Mom was the one who worried about everything, I was the one who questioned everything. I wasn't rebellious but maybe a little sassy. Why were things the way they were? I was always so curious and was never satisfied with the answer: "It's just the way it is." For example, Mom was from an era when the women and girls cared for the men and the boys in the home. "God made them the very same way he made me, Mom," I'd often argue, not wanting to assume this role. I determined early on to break that pattern in my own life and in my own family one day.

When Mom was in the hospital near the end of her life, she finally admitted to me that she had worried far more than was necessary. I think part of the reason why she died early was that she worried herself needlessly. "Don't be like me, whatever you do," she told me, lying in her hospital bed one day. I knew what she meant because she had often told us, "If you're going to worry, don't pray. And if you're going to pray, don't worry." Mom was a woman of great faith and believed that truth with her whole heart, but she could not turn off the anxiety. She felt tremendously responsible for everything and everyone. More people can relate to Mom than you would ever believe. They may appear to be calm on the outside, but inside they are a mess of nerves and consumed with anxiety. I see it in my clinic every day.

Growing up free in the fields of our farm and within the relative safety of our small town, I learned there was a choice: live and enjoy life in the moment, or be overcome by sadness and ill health. Let go and let God, or worry yourself to death. If you learned to make the right choice, it seemed to me from an early age that you would be just fine, and all the things you were tempted to worry about would work out eventually. Later when I was an adult studying anatomy and physiology as part of my training, my mom's tendency to worry came to mind. I wondered what effect constant worry had had on her health, and I made a startling discovery. The books I was reading said it wasn't just a bad idea to be anxious. Negative thoughts that consume our minds actually have a damaging physical effect on our bodies. Our cells change shape when we continually give in to anxiety. They don't smooth out and instead resemble circles with chips taken out of the edges. These misshapen cells clunk around in the body. The end result of self-induced stress is that you increase your propensity for disease and eventually get ill. All from worry.

There are things we can do to reduce worry. I'll repeat what Mom would say, "If you're going to worry, don't pray. If you're going to pray, don't worry." It is most certainly a choice. One option will drive you to your grave fast, and the other may lighten your loafers a little bit. Sometimes the best place to start when you want to let it all go is what I often did on the farm: open the door, get outside, and just look up.

I often remind the practitioners at my clinic, "Go outside and look up when you get home from work." We look down all day at bodies on tables, and our focus is so narrow because we're concentrating on our work to perform the best job possible. Office workers have the same problem, staring at a computer screen all day. At the end of the day, we all have to remember to raise our heads to the wondrous sky above and take a good, long look. We all need to expand our view when it comes to seeing the bigger picture in life. If we don't do that, we will keep our tiny world confined to only what we see before us, leaving little to no room for other thoughts.

I love to run, always have. When I'm on my outings with my trusty lab, Scout, we watch people on the trails. Every run is different, but something is almost always the same.

Very few are looking at the world around them. Where are their eyes turned? Most people we pass are absolutely laser-focused on one thing: their feet. If something goes wrong with their shoes, they'll know it immediately. It's so hard for me to pass them and not say, "Hey, you—look around! Look how beautiful this day is!" When I'm running, I know where my feet are at all times so I won't trip, but I do look around me. So does Scout. It makes our run go faster, and it helps my attitude to appreciate how beautiful my surroundings are in the woods of Prescott, Arizona.

Mom wasn't the only one who prioritized health in our family. Dad placed a similar focus on it, especially when it came to his animals. Although farming and agriculture underwent several technical advancements at that time, my father didn't routinely use anything artificial in the care of his animals, even when it would benefit him to do so. While some neighbors practiced artificial insemination to make life easier, Dad refused to do it. If one of his animals was sick, he would isolate it and just let the bug run its course. If the cow needed antibiotics, he would administer it (while keeping the animal away from the rest of the herd) and dump the milk after milking her until she was healthy again. He never trough-fed his calves because that could lead to pneumonia, but he recruited his children to bottle-feed each one instead, which took hours of additional time every day.

I was in charge of all the baby calves and took care of feeding them. Dad showed me how to do it and then turned the job over to me. There was an expectation that once you were taught well and had no questions, you should just go do it. Many of my clients comment that I have very strong fingers, and I tell them it's from years of bottle-feeding calves. I placed the nipple between my index and middle finger and grasped the one-gallon bottle with my ring finger, pinky, and thumb. When a calf latched on, I had to hang on with all my strength even when my hands ached. One spring we had 37 Holstein baby calves. These black-and-white cows tend to have similar patterns, and it was hard to keep track of which ones I'd fed because they would all crowd up around me. To remedy the situation, I took a red magic marker and numbered them 1-37 on the middle of their forehead. Dad often commented how most people think of cattle as unintelligent animals, and yet they're anything but. I called my calves by number, and they learned their number in a short time. I usually fed two calves at once, repeating this process twice a day!

I was the youngest girl and four years younger than the next sister in line. Several of my four sisters were out of the house by the time I graduated high school. So I grew up a tomboy running barefoot in the woods and fields with my two brothers. My baby brother, Dean, and I are just a year and a few months apart. Dean and I love to share stories about how often the three of us would get into trouble, or get hurt. Dean was always a thinker who carefully considered his ways before launching out. I was a little more daring. And Daryl was off the charts.

Michigan summers are beautiful with warm, sunny days and comfortable nights. Winter is a different story, with an average snowfall of several feet every season, so we had a lot of fun in the snow. One particularly snowy winter, Dad used his tractor to push a mound of snow into a pile near the milk house, and we kids quickly made it into a toboggan hill. As usual, it was Daryl who challenged me, along with Dean, to climb up into the haymow, make our way onto the roof of the milk house, and slide down the pile of snow.

When we got bored of that, we talked our dad into taking us tobogganing down another nearby hill that was much bigger than the one Dad made at the milk house. Dad drove us to the hill in his pickup truck, parked on the side of the road, and we set off into the woods carrying the toboggan high above our heads.

I was 10, and Daryl and I were the only daredevils willing to sled down the hill while the others agreed to watch from a safe distance. Our first pass was successful, although we jumped off the toboggan halfway down when it got too scary. It was so much fun that we walked back up for one more ride, and this time we intended to grit our teeth and make it all the way to the bottom.

I was sitting in the front of the toboggan with my legs out straight in front of me, trying to steer (eyes tightly shut) as Daryl held on in back. Bits of the fine, powdery snow blasted us in the face the whole way until suddenly I didn't feel any snow on my cheeks. I opened my eyes at that moment and discovered we were airborne.

We landed so hard it knocked the wind out of me. Daryl just laughed and grabbed my arm to yank me back up on my feet. But I could not stand up. I had no pain and wasn't crying, so neither of us initially realized the seriousness of the situation.

Looking back, I understand that my body was probably in shock from the hard crash. Daryl called me a baby and told me to get up. Patience was not his strong suit, and it's not mine either. I reached down and could not feel my legs. When I told him that I couldn't move, my brother rolled his eyes and said that I'd just ruined the day. Daryl yelled to tell our dad that something had happened to me.

Dad hurried down, and I will never forget the look in my father's eyes. He told me not to move then knelt down in the snow and instructed me very calmly that he was going to put me on his back while I held onto his neck. Dad stood up, and I held on tightly while my legs dangled helplessly underneath me. I felt Daryl's hand on the small of my back as he helped Dad up the steep hill.

Dad situated us in the back of the pickup, and the rest of my worried siblings held tightly onto me during the bumpy ride. Dad carried me into the house, laid me on the living room floor, and placed his warm, familiar hands on my neck. My mom, nervously wiping her hands on her apron, came out of the kitchen to ask what he thought was wrong with me.

He said nothing at first before informing her that we needed to go to the hospital immediately. "I'm pretty sure she's broken her back," I heard him whisper to my mom.

But he'd never touched my back. He only touched my neck. How could he know that with just a simple touch? I was destined to learn much more about the incredible power of human touch, and I was blessed to encounter it at such a young age from someone I loved and trusted.

Over the next few hours at the hospital, doctors told me

that I would never walk again. Never run. Never play. And never have children. The word "never" reverberated inside the stark white room of the hospital. It was a word I would come to dislike and one I learned to avoid saying to anyone else.

2

the colorful tour

THE DOCTORS WANTED to do surgery because they thought I'd fractured L2 and L3 (the second and third vertebrae in the lumbar spine). The risk was that this injury could leave me paralyzed, which is why they felt I would never run, never have children, all these "nevers." I remember Mom reached over and covered my ears so I wouldn't hear their drastic prognosis as I laid on the gurney after the X-rays.

When the doctors left us by ourselves to discuss our options privately, Mom bent down and told me, "Listen here, young lady. You *will* run again. You *will* have children when you're old enough. You *will* heal."

If Mom said so, I knew I'd be fine. Dad had news for the doctors when they returned to hear what we had decided as a family. "No surgery," he informed them. He had a better idea. "Put Lynell in traction instead. She's 10—she'll heal."

Despite the doctors' wishes, the hospital put me in

traction for one month just as Dad wanted. I laid perfectly still for four weeks, flat on my back. When I came home from the hospital on Christmas Day, I wore an uncomfortable brace that helped space apart the discs in my spinal cord in order to take pressure off my lumbar spine.

While I continued recovering, I could not sit or stand upright without that brace, and I wore it faithfully for about a year until I was strong again. Every morning, I would ring a bell on my bedside table to alert Mom so she could help me get out of bed and stand up. I missed out on so much of my classwork in the spring that Mom ended up tutoring me until I could return to the classroom for the last few weeks of the schoolyear before summer break.

We had a round above-ground swimming pool behind our home, and I spent the rest of the summer months rehabbing in it. Mom never learned how to swim, but she bravely waded into the water with me all summer. We held hands as we slowly and carefully made our way around in a circle. When I was stronger, she was much more comfortable standing guard outside the pool and walking with me around the edge, still tightly holding onto my hand.

Dad was right. I healed. And everything the doctors said I would never do, Mom made sure I did. I played with my brothers in the woods and even ran track in middle school. My injury didn't hold me back from anything I wanted to do. Eventually, just as Mom predicted, this too passed, and I went on to high school.

Mom could be counted on to share her ideas for all of us to consider when planning our lives. But in high school

I truly didn't know what I wanted to do after graduation. I had already disappointed her early on because I couldn't see myself doing the only two things she thought her second youngest child should pursue: becoming a teacher or a doctor. I didn't have the patience for teaching kids, and I definitely didn't like bodily fluids. All my brothers and sisters followed my mom's career advice, and they turned out fine. I, however, found it difficult to settle on just one path for the rest of my life. For a naturally curious person who asks questions about why things are the way they are, there were so many things out there in the world for me to learn.

Thankfully, life has a way of surprising us along the way. My current career in bodywork is something I stumbled into when I was busy being a wife and mom pursuing a totally different field. That's how it's been my entire life—being guided along the way, even when it seemed as if there was no plan in place. Even my experience being nearly paralyzed as a child would come full circle much later when I discovered my calling: helping put injured bodies back together. There would be a greater purpose to that struggle far in the future when someone special would come to my clinic out of the blue and ask me for help. In turn, he would teach me so much about the resilience of the human body—and the strength of the human spirit.

I floated between the popular crowd and not-so-popular kids who were more on the sidelines in high school. I could get along with anyone, but I spent most of my time with three close girlfriends. They knew exactly what they wanted to do after graduation and didn't seem to mind that I didn't have a clue. One of my friends named Krista was adamant about being a Marine from the time she was a freshman. A recruiter came to our school one day, and she was hooked. But I had no desire to volunteer for the unique privilege of having someone yell at me and tell me what to do all day. No way. Stacey wanted to join the Air Force, and that's what she did until she retired and became a realtor. Renee, the third friend, didn't want to go to college. She just wanted to be a mom, and that's what she ended up doing. Me? I look back on that time and jokingly say that I did the colorful tour.

I graduated high school with no particular plans whatsoever. I left home at 18 and never returned except to visit. I went to Western Michigan University for no other reason than I had to get my core classes out of the way. I spent two years there treading water and eventually decided that I might as well go into social work since I liked people. In one of my classes I had to volunteer at a shelter for physically abused women. That experience was supposed to be an internship of sorts, but the whole social worker career went wrong after I ended up rescuing a woman three times from the same man who was intent on beating her up.

Each time she went back to her abuser, I grew more confused by her behavior. She was a mom, and I could not understand why she was making such bad decisions for her family. In the infinite wisdom that only a 19-year-old thinks they have, I thought she was simply being foolish. But I was probably the foolish one in some respects. I often accompanied the police on domestic calls at this woman's house, putting myself in danger. This pattern happened repeatedly, but I am not a fearful person in any sense of the word, so I did not think anything of it at the time.

One night I caught her in the women's shelter kitchen talking softly on the phone with her husband. She wasn't supposed to have any contact with the guy. I immediately took the phone away from her and hung up the receiver. I don't know where I got the strength to do it because that degree of boldness is normally not part of my personality.

I told her, "If you want to go back to him, go back. But your kids are staying here in this shelter. They don't need to see you do this. Do you want to keep the cycle of abuse going? Is that your plan?"

The woman was looking at me, wild-eyed and saying nothing. The director of the shelter happened to walk in while I had this conversation and informed me privately later, "I don't think this work is for you." She was right.

Even at that young age I could not tolerate stupidity. I was furious that the lady we were trying to help was hurting her kids. The shelter didn't need to fire me—I was just a volunteer anyway. There was no way I was going to do that job, I told myself. But I had to come up with some other plan for my future. So I moved to Grand Rapids to continue my education in a bigger city. I worked two jobs while I attended class and earned my associate degree in Liberal Arts at Grand Rapids Community College. Whoop tee doo, I remember thinking when I stared at my diploma. Oh well, at least I got something.

Then one day on a lark I registered for electrical engineering at ITT Tech after seeing a pamphlet about it. I loved it immediately, and my grades showed that I had developed a passion for something for the first time in my educational journey thus far. The work reminded me of unwinding the chains of necklaces when I was a kid. I loved to dig through a jewelry box, find the biggest knotted wad of gold chains, and slowly take the time to unravel each one. That level of tedium drove other people nuts, but to me it was relaxing. At ITT Tech the circuit boards and connecting of wires made sense to me. I had phenomenal instructors, was the only girl in my class, and was 4.0'ing it.

Mom saw the change in me and casually remarked that I had always been good with my hands, often spending free time on the farm as a kid fixing small electronics like transistor radios. She encouraged me to continue studying electrical engineering, complete my degree, and possibly get a job in that field.

"You won't know until you try," she urged me.

I had energy to spare and kept myself occupied outside of class by working at Target as a cashier at night and holding down a day job at Foremost Insurance Company in their payroll department. I was soon promoted to the accounts receivable department at Foremost where I worked with insurance agents all over the country. I was barely 20 years old, and despite my young age I quickly assumed the responsibility of managing several large accounts for the company.

Anyone who grew up on a farm can multi-task as naturally as they can breathe. It was nothing for me to balance half a dozen chores at once. Working in a busy office environment didn't seem that different to me. I earned good money, but I was bored to death trapped inside the four empty walls of my cubicle all day, daydreaming of something else I could do to support myself.

The best thing about my job at the insurance company is that I met my future husband, Pete. We'd talked briefly once at work when he stopped by my desk to introduce himself. Then another co-worker invited him to join us for drinks after work. I had to study later for an engineering class exam, so I was about to leave when he finally showed up. Pete and I ended up talking until the place closed. Although I never got to study, I aced my exam. We were engaged six months later when I was 23 years old.

When I married Pete, I ended up dropping out of my engineering classes because my focus had changed, and I was ready for a new adventure. When we got married, the priest gave us what he called the "best advice" he gives to all young married couples. He told us to move 1,000 miles away from both sets of parents for the first year because it forces you to depend on each other. I desperately wanted to experience life outside of the Midwest, something I'd dreamed of doing for as long as I could remember. My husband put in for a transfer with the insurance company, and I looked forward to getting out of Michigan and spreading my wings. Still, Michigan would always have my heart because our families are back there, and today I'm the only one of my six siblings who still lives so far away.

My parents were not happy at all when we moved two

thousand miles away to Mesa, Arizona, in 1992. It wasn't my favorite location either, and I wasn't much happier when my husband transferred to Las Vegas a year later. But we grew up a lot during our time in the desert. We were learning to be married and rely on each other in many ways. The first year I also learned to cook for two. Pete was kind to eat more than one serving at every meal, which helped me adjust the portions. Vegas would be the last time I made our home in the dry desert, yet it wouldn't be my last visit to the Southwest. Of course, I did not know that at the time.

I got a job in administration working for a family in Vegas who owned a development company working the area around Black Mountain, an iconic mountain south of the Las Vegas valley. Then I got pregnant, and the owners were so wonderful to me. There was a large-scale criminal operation kidnapping blonde-haired, blue-eyed children in the Vegas area around that time, so I did not want to put my young daughter in daycare or hire a stranger to watch her at our home while my husband and I worked. The owners agreed to give me eight months of paid time off so I could be at home with my newborn baby. They were phenomenal people, and I've never forgotten the generosity they showed our young family. My husband transferred again to Georgia before I could return to work.

Pete, our daughter, and I moved to the Deep South where we lived for five terrific years. That was probably one of my favorite places, raising a family and living amid the farmland and mountains. That's also where I resurrected my engineering interests and started a new job working for an engineering firm called Siemens Energy and Automation. I was back in the complex electrical, mechanical, and chemical world that I loved, and I felt very fulfilled in my new role in their human resources department.

Although I never earned my B.A. in Engineering, I understood enough about the electrical engineering portion of the business that I could put those puzzles together and work well with the engineers. Even though I lacked a formal degree in the field, I interviewed well, and Siemens ended up providing on-the-job training. I love learning and earned multiple certifications in human resources. Looking back, this opportunity was a perfect match with my personality.

In fact, I could see myself building a long-term career working for Siemens. That was a new feeling for me. But something was going on back home in Michigan that would soon disrupt those plans and eventually change the trajectory of my entire life.

I received a call from Dad one evening and learned that Mom was very sick. I immediately booked a ticket from Georgia to Michigan to see my parents and ended up staying several weeks to care for her. All the children took turns helping Dad take care of Mom. She was experiencing renal failure, which eventually led to a kidney transplant. Her brother volunteered to be her donor, and I drove them from Michigan to Wisconsin for the procedure. After her recovery, it was not a difficult decision to pack up our home in Georgia and move back to Michigan when it was obvious Mom needed more help. It was an extra advantage that Pete could transfer again with Foremost, and the move put us closer to Pete's family as well.

We rented a house about five miles from the hospital where Mom was receiving care. However, that was an hour drive from home where Dad continued doing his best to hold down the farm and the endless responsibilities there. Because I lived so close to the hospital, it was my phone that rang in the middle of the night when there was a problem, but I did not mind. More than once, I got dressed and drove in the dark to see Mom and talk with the nurses.

Michigan is one of the prettiest states in the Midwest, and it felt right to be there again after being away so many years. I landed a job with another engineering company in their HR department, while Pete stayed busy working at Foremost and helping his parents and siblings develop some family property that we planned to build on one day. The property was large and had been handed down through generations of his mom's family. Pete was working on a strategy to use it to help support his parents in their older years. He was concerned about his own mom and dad's wellbeing, because that's the way he is. All his siblings had an opportunity to buy some of the land at a discount, and our portion was absolutely gorgeous with rolling green hills and mature trees dotting the landscape. There was a gully running down the middle, and wildflowers like Jack in the Pulpit and Lady Slippers lined its banks. I didn't know the names of these flowers, but Pete's mom did. She walked the property with us and told us about her memories growing up there.

I picked out the perfect house plans one day while thumbing through dozens of old issues of *Country Living* magazine stacked in my mother-in-law's living room. I always flipped through those magazines whenever we visited her, and my eyes were drawn to a sketch of the ideal home for our tract of land. I could picture us living there for many years, family all around us, in a place we could finally call our own and settle down.

Meanwhile, my mom's health inevitably deteriorated from 1999 to 2001. Just before she passed away, our family took turns sitting with Mom around the clock at the hospital. One day I was sitting beside her bed massaging her feet, waiting for Dad to arrive and relieve me. She had been sleeping more as her time drew near, and I was used to the quiet hours that passed as I sat with her. Suddenly, she made a motion as if she were trying to sit up in the bed. I was startled to see her move her body because she'd had no energy for so long. Then she spoke.

"You have your father's hands, Lynell," she told me in a voice that was much stronger than I anticipated. "You have to do something with those hands."

I laughed, not knowing if this was the medication talking. "I am doing something, can't you feel this?" I said, squeezing both of her heels.

That's when she wagged her finger in a way that I'd seen her do a thousand times in my lifetime and said, "Listen here, young lady...you'll get it one of these days."

Dad walked in at that moment, and I told him what had

just happened. We both agreed that it was likely the drugs influencing her, and I left him alone with Mom and went home.

It was the last conversation I had with my mom. The doctors put her back on the ventilator, and she died a few days later. It was a cold November day in 2001 the day I told her goodbye for the last time.

Mom died, and a seed was planted for something new to begin. Life is like that. Something passes on, and something new begins. This "something new" began on that last day I saw Mom alive when Pete and I were in the elevator on the way up to see her. We were quiet when suddenly he said, "I have the weird feeling we're going to move again."

"Nope," I said with finality. I did not even want to consider that prospect at that moment. Pete was fortunate to retain his work with Foremost Insurance for most of his career, and they had moved him around the country when they had openings. In years past, I'd always just rolled with it whenever Pete changed jobs. I was always the one who would have to get a new job wherever we landed. I would start over once more with new friends and try to make the most of it, no matter what happened. Honestly, I enjoyed the adventure up to a point. Not this time. We had been living in Michigan for nearly three years. I couldn't bear to think about uprooting our lives again and all the stressful decisions that would have to be made, including finding a new elementary school for our young daughter. I knew we'd have to go down the familiar house shopping route, and I'd have to interview for yet another job. The list went on and on, and I knew each step very well.

Pete did not even have a job offer somewhere else at the time. It was just a feeling he had about our future. I turned to him as the doors opened on the hospital elevator and said, "If there is one blip …one hurdle to jump over…I'm not moving anywhere." If we were going to leave our families behind again, I wanted it to be the easiest move we'd ever made, or else I was planning to dig in my heels.

We didn't talk about it for a while after that because our hearts were heavy with grief over losing my mom. But Pete's hunch about our future came to fruition a few months later when he had an opportunity in the spring of 2002 to move to the Southwest with Foremost. Fortunately, by the time the subject of moving away from Michigan came up again, I had softened a little. But I still didn't want to move. Instead of flat out refusing to go, I now proposed that the only way I would go is if the new house had a pool and a piano.

There was a claims position opening in the Arizona region with Foremost, and Pete was offered a choice between living up north in Prescott or down south in Phoenix or Tucson. He would be working out of the house and going out on the road pretty much all the time either way. The decision between the two cities was obvious, we agreed, after Pete and I visited Prescott. In contrast to the dry heat and desert of Phoenix and Tucson, Prescott is over 5,000 feet above sea level in the Prescott National Forest. It has all four seasons in a mild form, including warm summers and cold winters with an occasional layer of snow. Prescott is also a small town, and it felt like a better fit for us after growing up the way we both did in Michigan.

I had just had surgery on both feet when we went on our scout trip to see how we would like living in Arizona. I had bad bunions and a phenomenal surgeon in Michigan who was not keen on doing the correction on both feet at the same time. But because I ran and did kick-boxing and was very active, in addition to working full time, I wasn't going to be put down for 12 weeks recovering at home. I figured my body was strong enough, so I talked him into killing two birds with one stone. I wasn't supposed to put a lot of weight on my feet, so we did a lot of driving around on that trip. The landscape of Northern Arizona was not as vivid and green as I would have liked, and the unusual beauty of the Southwest was no match for Michigan, in my opinion. But it had its pluses, and I finally resigned myself to the fact that we would move there. Looking back, I can see that it was a good thing that my husband was more open to moving from the beginning. Or else I would have missed out on so much.

Pete ended up moving first to start his new job, while I stayed in Michigan to pack up and finish out the schoolyear with our daughter. For weeks he tried to find a home for sale with a pool, a rare feature in Prescott because of the mild weather. That man worked his butt off trying to make that happen for me. He even called me in desperation one night and asked if a place with a community pool would be acceptable.

"No, I'm not sharing," I assured him.

Well, he asked, would I be willing to compromise if he found a place with a piano and enough room to build a pool? I agreed.

While Pete was house hunting, I began doing a little bit of research about what I could do and where I could work in that area of the country. This was long before it was so easy to search online. The Internet was not packed full of information in 2002 like it is today. Human resources would be a natural place for me to start looking for jobs, but my mom's last words kept coming to mind. "You need to do something with those hands…"

We didn't have a computer at home. So the day before I left my office for the final time, something prompted me to search "work with hands." All kinds of massage and chiropractic links came up on the screen. Then I saw at the bottom of the search results something about Bowtech Technique. I clicked on that link and quickly learned that Bowtech was a specific type of bodywork that originated in Australia. I saw Tom Bowen's name as the founder, and I presumed it had been named after him.

There wasn't a ton of information on the website, but I read with interest a list that stated what this technique was and, more important, what it wasn't. That list resonated with me for some reason. I was relieved because it said it wasn't fascia work, and it wasn't massage. None of that interested me because I don't have a great stomach for bodily fluids or hairy backs. But what piqued my interest was that it seemed to describe the nervous system in electrical terms. I read over the list quickly one more time, and then tucked it away in the back of my mind. I never forgot it. Call it a blessing or a curse, I don't often forget much.

At the end of the summer, my daughter and I headed

south and joined Pete in Prescott. It was difficult to leave my family and all the dreams we'd been building for our future in Michigan, but my conversation with Pete in the elevator at the hospital helped reassure me that we were probably doing the right thing. I had insisted on a smooth transition if we moved, and the process had gone forward exactly like that—without a hitch. Not one blip! The house my husband found came with a piano, and true to his word, he put a pool in the backyard! I have always loved the green landscape of Michigan, and truthfully there was not enough of that for me in my new home. But I learned to appreciate the wide-open spaces of Prescott, and if I had to leave Lake Michigan behind, at least our family pool brought me somewhat near water!

We still live in this same home today, and have made so many memories here as a family. Sometimes when I'm alone relaxing or exercising in the pool, my mind drifts back to those days when Mom bravely donned her swimsuit and hopped in the water with me when I was a child. She must have been terrified since she couldn't swim, but her love for me overrode her fear.

It's funny how life works out the way it's supposed to. If Mom had not gotten sick, we probably would have stayed in Georgia the rest of our lives. But there was a great big reason why we moved to Prescott after Mom died, and I would spend the next few years finding out exactly what that reason was. And when I did discover it, no one would be more surprised than me.

I took three weeks to unpack once we arrived in Arizona, including painting our daughter's room to make her feel at home in our new place. I created an entire jungle on her bedroom walls. I didn't know I could do that. I painted a wild scene with all kinds of animals, including a Zebra drinking from a pond and even added a tree as a canopy over her bed, with stars peeking through the leaves.

When we registered our daughter for school, we met her teachers and ran into some other parents one afternoon. One of the fathers was a big German man named Klaus. We were doing the usual small talk thing, chatting about our kids, when he asked what Pete did for a living. Then he asked me where I worked. I was about to say I had a background in HR when I heard myself give a completely different answer. I told Klaus how I had read about the Bowtech Technique and wanted to learn how to become a practitioner. It just popped right out of my mouth! Pete cast a curious glance over at me but said nothing.

Then it was my turn to be surprised when Klaus said, "Is that right? Hold on a second. Let me get something for you that you might be interested in."

He fished in his pocket for his wallet, pulled out a business card, and handed it to me. "I'm not sure if this is what you're talking about," he said, "but I just met this lady the other day."

On the card was a name and her title, "Bowtech Technique Instructor," underneath. I was taken aback by what seemed like a weird coincidence. Klaus explained that he was training to be a medical masseuse and was also interested in learning about this technique. Furthermore, Klaus told us that the lady on the business card had just moved to Prescott herself three weeks before we did.

Normally, I am a private person. I generally don't engage strangers with my personal history, but I found myself telling Klaus that I had a background in the corporate world and zero experience in bodywork. He didn't laugh when I confessed that, only commenting off-handedly about maybe it being time for a change. Something in me needed to hear that small affirmation, even if it was from someone I did not know. I took a few days to think about this odd and unplanned encounter. I wasn't sure if I should call the instructor's phone number on the card or not.

What made much more sense was sending in my resume to Wulfsberg Electronics after I saw an ad in the paper for a job opening in their human resources department. That is what I *should* do, I reminded myself. So I sent my resume to Wulfsberg and then picked up the phone to call the bodywork instructor!

I introduced myself and told her about my interest in learning, but she didn't want to teach me. And she was pretty blunt about it. I can't blame her. After all, I was about as far away from pursuing bodywork as someone with my lack of experience could get. I was a corporate junkie—a hard and fast HR worker with a long history in traditional employment who was used to hiring and firing people, not healing them. It was laughable when you think about it, and my inquiry must have come across as quite a bold proposal.

I had to bug this instructor for eight weeks just to take me seriously. "I'm supposed to learn this," I told her in one of our subsequent phone calls. "I know I am." I didn't know *why* I was supposed to learn it. There was simply a deep knowing inside of me, and that's all I had to go on. "Just tell me what I need to do and what classes I need to take, and I will do it." This path was meant to be, and I felt it with everything inside of me.

In all that time, I never told Pete about what I was doing. I usually let stuff tumble around in my head like clothes in a dryer until I'm secure in how I feel about it before I open my mouth. When the instructor finally gave in to my persistence and agreed to let me sit in on the next evening class, I told Pete what was happening. By this time, I had already interviewed and accepted the job at Wulfsberg working in their HR department.

After I explained everything, I said, "Can't you see Mom standing next to God and telling him to put me here in Prescott right now?" I was laughing as I thought about Mom informing God how to help her easily-distracted child who had happily wandered aimlessly for years up to this point. There was no other way to explain this sudden left turn in my career other than the fact that Someone was guiding me.

When I arrived for my first class, there were three other students. The instructor had a way of teaching that made learning memorable and fun. The context of this kind of unique bodywork is incredibly detailed in medical science, and I guarantee I had never even heard of the terms and techniques she was talking about during that first class. Nevertheless, what I learned that night clicked with me at once. It made sense, and I longed to learn more.

As I furiously took notes, I told myself, "I'm going to put bodies back together." This opportunity excited and energized me to the core of my being. I got in my car and flew home that night, anxious to tell my husband that I had stumbled onto something I wanted to do for the rest of my life. I just had to figure out how to make that happen.

3

giving the body its due

I CONTINUED WORKING in HR at the engineering company to earn a steady income and took bodywork classes after work and on weekends. One day a co-worker at Wulfsberg fell on the job and came to my office to complete routine paperwork for a workplace injury. She had worn high heels to work that day and twisted her ankle. It was swollen like a balloon, and her back was hurting. She was in quite a bit of pain, describing her symptoms to me as I wrote up the incident report. While she was talking, I thought to myself that I knew how to fix her. Then I told her how I was learning body and nerve restoration techniques and asked if she wanted me to try a little something.

With her consent, I laid her on the floor and worked on her using the few moves I'd learned in class so far. We were both smiling when the swelling went down within five minutes. It wasn't just like putting on an ice pack. The immediate difference was as obvious as it was shocking. I was floored, and so was she. Word spread like wildfire throughout the office about what I was learning.

When I initially discovered this technique, I pursued it for the simple reason that I wanted to help people. I was familiar with massage as a type of bodywork, but I could see right away that what I was learning was different. I'm a fixer by nature, so I need to get down to the nitty gritty to find out why something is not working, which is what this technique does. Plus, it didn't hurt to learn that clients remain fully clothed for their session, unlike massage!

We knew very few people in Prescott when I began training to become a Bowen practitioner, because we had not had time to make any friends. We were both busy with our jobs, settling in, and raising a child. I initially practiced the bodywork techniques I was learning on the closest guinea pigs I could find, my husband and daughter. Then I began to see other people and other bodies in a different way. Instead of faintly noticing a person's clothes or the way they styled their hair, I saw a drooping shoulder, a stiff back, or a funny gait. If we were out in public shopping or eating in a restaurant, my eyes would intently focus on someone's ailment as my mind tried to work out exactly what was wrong with them. Sometimes I would walk up to a perfect stranger, introduce myself, and tell them I was learning a bodywork technique. Could I practice on them?

And they would just let me do it! I think I embarrassed my family more than once when I would stop someone on the sidewalk downtown on Prescott's courthouse square to try a move I'd just learned so I could see what it would do.

I progressed in my education and added pre-med anatomy and physiology to my studies, with a focus on the nervous system. I was thankful I'd had a teacher for a mom because she set the foundation for how to study and think critically. My instructor noticed I was a quick learner with an unusual aptitude for the material. She even began allowing me to work on clients who came to see her if she did not have time. Meanwhile, I also enrolled in an online college to study Holistic Nutrition and completed my undergraduate degree.

What ended up happening next was the opposite of what I ever intended. My future business career was born in Prescott that fall. My instructor had as much impact on getting my business started and building my reputation as my own initiative and willingness to practice on anyone who would let me. I worked out of my house before I received my official certification and slowly began building my future clientele. Although I could not charge people while I waited to be certified, my instructor reminded me that I was well-trained and should never work for free.

If you offer something for free, it doesn't matter what it is, no one puts any stock in it. The same was true for my amateur status in bodywork. Although I loved it so much and would have worked on anyone for free, I followed my instructor's advice and made a rule that clients had to give something in exchange for my service. It could not be gratis. People gladly donated five dollars or something non-monetary like an apple or a bag of oranges.

Working out of my house went well at the start. Pete and

I shared office space downstairs, and the house was perfect because it has a separate entrance. I bought a couple of tables for clients and tried to make the setting as professional as possible. It was haphazard, but I had to make it work if I was going to make a living doing this. I was still working full-time for the engineering firm and scheduled clients after work in the evening. I tried to make appointments when Pete was out on the road, but one day I booked a few clients when he was home.

Around dinnertime, two people were on the tables relaxing in la la land, and my husband put a pizza in the oven, since he would be on his own for supper. Suddenly the smoke alarm started blaring, and our two dogs began howling at the top of their lungs, startling my clients awake and undoing every ounce of relaxation and healing I'd been creating for the past hour. Pete sat down to a burned pizza later that evening, and I made a big decision.

That was the night I started thinking seriously about moving my business out of the house and leasing space somewhere in town. If I was going to do this professionally and do it well, I told myself, I really shouldn't be doing it from my house while sharing space with a working husband, two dogs, and a cat.

I can't say that I always dreamed of being a business owner leading a staff of employees, but I've always been comfortable in a leadership role. I probably grew into that role naturally from watching Mom and Dad. He loved being a farmer and an entrepreneur. He never thought about our family farm as a small business, but it was. Mom skillfully steered a houseful of kids, and our small-town community also put her to work. She volunteered to run all the local school programs, so I had plenty of opportunities to learn from her what leadership looked like. Mom had a certain stature that convinced casual observers she was the leader without her having to take a stand or make a point. Everybody followed her inside and outside of our home. She was an educator, but I never saw Mom teach in a traditional classroom because by the time I was born she had retired to be a full-time mom.

When I started out as an entrepreneur, I wasn't a leader of anyone. Working alone out of a downstairs room in our home while I looked for office space to lease allowed me to eventually build up about 10 "regulars" who came to the house. I give credit to one of these early clients for changing the entire way I did business after working on him the first time.

At the end of the session, he got up from the table and started to leave. Then he asked, "So what do I do now?" I wasn't sure how to respond. So I thought for a long minute before I answered.

Being new at this venture, I wasn't prepared for that question. I personally don't like being told what to do. We were not raised that way by my parents—we were expected to think for ourselves. Do what your conscience tells you to do, my parents often said. If something is off that mark, they cautioned us, you'll know that you better not do it. I didn't have much of an inclination to tell others what to do with their health at this point.

"Do I come back to see you next week or what?" my client clarified, filling in the silence between us.

"Yes…if you want to," I told him casually, taking note of the dissatisfied look on his face regarding my non-committal answer. He left, and I kept replaying that scene in my mind the rest of the night.

Later that evening, I concluded that I was going to have to be a leader for my clients. Most people, I've since learned, don't mind being led. They're happier when they can follow the guidance of someone they trust—and trust the one they follow. Mom used to say that was the case, and I knew instinctively that night that she was right. I realized that I didn't want to just make people feel good and then send them home. They desperately needed to be guided along the way— but gently. When I started actively directing my clients' health journey, everything changed, including me. That one decision transformed the entire focus of my work, and the business absolutely skyrocketed from that point forward.

My original plan was to continue with my HR "real job" with a paycheck and benefits and get certified in bodywork to help people on the side. By no means did I foresee quitting a stable job to become self-employed. Nor did I imagine this side hustle growing exponentially at such a rapid rate. I didn't anticipate moving into a series of bigger offices with multiple employees and part-time receptionists. I certainly didn't see the day coming when I would have the opportunity to buy the building where Lynell & Company houses the Body and

Nerve Restoration Center today.

All those dreams were still a long way off. The first step was moving from our home into my first office space. When I walked inside the rental unit, the walls were as black as a velvety night sky. The only window was crusty and sealed tight after years of accumulated dirt and neglect. It was winter in Prescott and the temperature was in the mid-forties, but there was no central heating. There was no air-conditioning either, and did I mention no hot water in the tap? I took a few steps on the uneven cement floors. The place was incredibly small, kind of haunted house creepy, and all mine. I signed the lease and felt a surge of pride as I held the keys in my hand. My first professional office space.

Dad loaned me $3000 start-up money, and I promised to pay it back in one-and-a-half years. If I couldn't make a profit in that time, I might as well give up and go back to corporate America, I told him. The landlord liked me and allowed me to put only a little money down and go month-to-month on the rent payments. I had a sense that Mom was probably lovingly suggesting from heaven behind the scenes that God make it easy for me and keep me focused.

Through a referral, I also eventually gained a business advisor in a sweet lady named Cynthia. She was a former professor at Yavapai College teaching entrepreneurship and a highly trained accountant. Cynthia talked to me about everything from business planning to taxes in rapid fire instructions and made her (excellent) opinions known. Left to my own devices, I would have helped anyone in pain and never asked for anything in return. That's how I am. Cynthia straightened me out.

"It is human nature to give everything away," she explained. "But you are not going to do that, because you will not make any money. You at least want to pay off your schooling, don't you?" She suggested I should have a receptionist to greet people because it would provide a buffer between me and clients.

I didn't have money to hire staff then, so I put my eight-year-old daughter and my best friend Karen's daughter at the front window. Analise and Cortney were so small that they shared the same office chair. Cortney was good with filing, and Analise proved to be good with the money. Both girls had great people skills. I broke all kinds of child labor laws using eight-year-olds as receptionists to greet people and answer the phones, but it got us off the ground.

I got to know the young tanning salon owners next door to my office who played loud pop music non-stop. They were trying to make the work hours go faster by cranking up the volume, but my clients were trying to relax! We worked out a code of three bangs on the wall whenever I needed them to turn down their music.

I coated every wall, including the front door, with a thick lavender paint to make the meager surroundings cheerier. To this day, people still talk about that purple front door. It's my favorite color, and purple communicated the soothing and relaxing environment I wanted. That unique door also served as free advertising and a reference point for new people to find us in town. My clients would tell their friends and co-workers, "Go see Lynell with the purple door." For three years until 2006, I worked at that office six days a week, eight to ten hours a day. Building a business often took me away from my family because I worked long days and many nights. (And still do today!) When our daughter was in school and Pete was traveling, I would work during the day, but then invariably someone would get hurt after hours. I scheduled clients in the evenings who worked 9-5 during the day. More of my personal time was sacrificed, but that was okay with me. Pete and I weren't raised to be travelers and take vacations—we didn't take one together for 18 years! We took day trips, but I never left the business overnight.

I built my clientele slowly and tenuously, hoping for the best but not entirely sure I could make it. It eventually became obvious that I had connected with what I was meant to do for the rest of my life. Once I knew that, my business shifted into another gear, and I never looked back.

Years earlier when I was a young mom working full-time in the corporate world, I longed to be in charge of my own schedule. That way, when my daughter was older, I could go to her games or take her to dance lessons. Early in our marriage I told Pete, "By the time Analise is 10, I will have my own business." I said it aloud as if it was a done deal. I remember my husband's blue eyes widened.

"And what job would that be?" he asked.

"I don't know yet, but I'll figure it out."

I had the business up and running by the time she was 8 years old. Today I'm in my eighteenth year of my side hustle, and my "real job" in HR is a distant memory. When you say something out loud, there is a greater likelihood that it will happen. Words can give life or suck it right out of a dream. I overheard some guys once say someone is either a Negative Nancy or Positive Pearl! When I heard myself set this goal of owning my business, it stuck with me—even though I had no idea then what business I wanted to start. That's how powerful the human brain can be. It's the same way with what we do in our clinic; the body and the mind work together as a team.

People often ask me, "What is it exactly that you do in your clinic?" The simplest way to say it is that our work is powered by the moves of Bowenwork. At its core, Bowen is a dynamic system of muscle and connective tissue therapy developed by the late founder, Tom Bowen, in Geelong, Australia. The technique has evolved because people were slower paced in his day, especially in rural Australia where he lived and worked. Today people are running like rats in a tin can, and the Internet and social media direct much of our lives. Over the years I have adapted how we see the body and how we can best work with the body. I've adjusted accordingly but have not changed the substance of what Tom taught. Taking the foundational moves of Bowen, I've developed them into specific protocols helping a range of issues with the human body. When the body suffers an injury, the body compensates. The goal behind the work is to help the body put in its corrections instead of compensations. The body is phenomenal at compensating and will always take the path of least resistance. The same is true of how it puts in corrections—it doesn't have to go into compensation mode but can just as easily go into healing mode.

What we do in my clinic is neither derived from nor similar to any other hands-on modality like massage or chiropractic work. The basic principle behind it is the idea that the body and the mind work separately, yet together. When I began this business, I had no idea how many people were totally fearful, anxious, and stressed out by life—and their bodies were subsequently in pain. Somehow, one after the other, these folks managed to find their way to my clinic.

Anxiety and stress can take you down a very dark rabbit hole. It's hard to climb out of it because the experience changes the chemistry in your brain. Instead of having good serotonin levels, which keep you calm and happy (they are your happy hormones), your hormones deplete themselves and kick on your adrenals to correct the problem. The role of anxiety in disease and unwellness is huge. It can take you out. I always say that if you have God as your foundation, there is no reason to be fearful. He's got you one way or the other. Being fearful about the future and wondering, "What if? What if?" is common to the human experience, but it's never from God.

Living with anxiety is so pervasive that most of the people you meet day-to-day live in constant fight or flight mode—the physiological response our ancestors had whenever they met with danger in their environment. When they saw a saber-toothed tiger, for example, they experienced shortness of breath, a rapid heartrate, and a surge of adrenaline while trying to decide whether to stand their ground and fight—

or flee. The danger modern humans face is not a tiger but more likely a demanding boss at the office or a traffic jam on a six-lane freeway. Many people have what we call high-functioning anxiety. They are the cashiers at the supermarket, your kids' teachers, and your neighbors. You don't necessarily recognize that they are stressed because they have learned to hide it extremely well in order to function in society. People think being on their phone all the time, working long hours, and being constantly on the go is just normal, with no time for real relaxation.

No matter how good you are at hiding or ignoring your stress, the body eventually gets overwhelmed from the constant rush of adrenaline day after day. It's like an open faucet running all day long. Remaining in this heightened fight or flight mode will inevitably lead to a breakdown physically or mentally.

I don't claim to be an expert who knows it all, but over the years I have worked on thousands of bodies, and from my earliest days I've seen a pattern in the clinic repeatedly. People have an emotional, physical, or mental imbalance—and/or they are chock full of anxiety and low-level fear that never quite goes away. The body, therefore, is out of whack because it's trying to compensate for the anxiety or imbalance that the person has accepted as part of their daily life. They don't even notice the lengths the body is going to, trying to compensate.

When we're anxious, the body must figure out a way to get through the day while having a proverbial "monkey" on its back. It's no wonder that clients come to the clinic complaining of numbness in their hands, a stiff back, clenched jaw, and the inability to turn their neck. All their stress is laying right on the tops of their shoulders.

"Are you feeling stressed?" I ask when they come in.

"No, not really," comes the response. "It's my daily life, you know." Meanwhile, it looks to me as if their ears are trying to attach to their shoulders because of all the stress they're carrying right there! I'm no exception. One of my practitioners tells me periodically when I've had a hard day, "Your ears don't need a shelf to sit on. Look in the mirror, Lynell!" I do, and I see that my right shoulder is clenched up to my ear, and I didn't even realize it.

I had a client who injured his back. We worked with him to input the corrections to address that issue, and it worked. One day he threw out his back while playing with his daughter in the pool. He remembered what I told him about stopping immediately if he ever felt his back go out again. He stopped and waited—right there in the pool. His body then took the past of least resistance, inputting corrections instead of starting down the path of compensation for another back injury. He felt several "clicks" and his back returned to a normal state in just a few minutes.

The body is amazing at making corrections and/or compensations, depending on the situation. Compensations come when we injure ourselves or do something (like stress ourselves out) where the body has to make a decision whether to compensate or correct. If we don't stop and give it a chance to "correct" what's wrong, then it has to compensate to keep us on the move. Had my client not stopped playing in the pool immediately, his body would have compensated for the injury to his back, instead of correcting it and taking the pain away.

Many people cannot remember the last time they took a deep breath. They are so anxious all the time that shallow breathing is normal. Consequently, some people may eventually feel as if they have allergies or low-grade asthma. In our clinic, we open the airways by performing a group of moves across the sternum into the Vagus nerve lines. We have the client take 10 deep breaths through the nose and out of the mouth, and in seconds the body re-trains itself to breathe deeply instead of compensating for constant shallow breathing. After this deep oxygenation to the brain and body, the client feels like a new person! They feel they can take on the world, and their head is clear for the first time in a long time. Deep breaths are the simplest first step to take toward healing.

The work we do helps the body to heal from several stress-related, continual compensation patterns and get it into a corrective pattern. Our job is to pull out the compensation (clenched jaws, tense shoulders, etc.) and put in the correction (restore and relax).

Rather than focusing on a single complaint, we address the entire body by restoring balance via the autonomic nervous system (ANS). The ANS controls over 80% of our bodily functions and is very susceptible to external stressors like jobs, relationships, etc. The ANS is further divided into two systems—sympathetic and parasympathetic. The sympathetic nervous system is what directs our body's involuntary response to stress. For example, we breathe harder and our heartrate speeds up. A cascade of hormones then washes over the body to increase blood flow and make us more alert and ready to fight the perceived danger.

In turn, the parasympathetic nervous system is responsible for calming us down after the crisis has passed. Our work operates on the belief that true healing can occur only after the ANS shifts from sympathetic (fight mode) to parasympathetic dominance (rest, relax, and repair mode). We do all we can to help clients make that shift.

As scientists do more research, they are finding that there are more nervous systems in the body than we've known about. It's kind of like the multiple universes they keep discovering in outer space in addition to the familiar one our little blue planet lives in. For example, there is also the enteric nervous system (ENS) that pertains to the gut, and here is where it gets even more interesting. The ENS is another one of the main divisions of the autonomic nervous system (ANS) and consists of a mesh-like system of neurons that controls the function of the gastrointestinal tract. It's an emotional nervous system that will analyze a situation and indicate that something is good or bad, right or wrong. So when you say you have a "gut feeling" about something or somebody, you're closer to the truth than you realize. The brain and spinal cord comprise the central nervous system (CNS), but the ENS is also called the second brain. It's derived from what are called neural crest cells (think: neurons in the brain).

I don't know which came first, the chicken or the egg, but we know that the enteric and central nervous systems develop at the same time through the umbilical cord. Based on that key knowledge, Tom Bowen said his goal with his work was to take the body back to where life began, where the nervous system began. The key in healing is to return the body back to its origin so it can reorganize itself to heal and return to a time of life without pain, without injury, without issue. We initiate our bodywork where it all began at the umbilical cord, and we expand outward from there.

The main thing to understand about how and why Bowen works is that the body and mind must work in sync together; when they are out of sync, problems arise. Because Bowen addresses the body as a whole unit, rather than just the presenting symptoms, the healing can occur at all levels as needed: physical, chemical, emotional, mental, energy-wise, and more. Sometimes called the homeopathy of bodywork, Bowen utilizes subtle inputs to the body through the hands, stimulating the body to heal itself, often profoundly.

Practitioners in our clinic are not there to tell the body what to do. They are merely well-trained facilitators. This makes Bowen unique from many other types of bodywork where the skill of the clinician is the focus. Instead, we give the body some direction, and then it chooses what it wants to do. Most of the time the body will choose to heal. Sometimes it will not, and we respect that.

Picture your body as a temple that houses your soul. We know our own bodies better than anyone because we're the ones living every day inside them! There is no janitorial staff for that temple—it's your job to keep that temple clean, orderly, and functioning. A team effort is required to heal (between a client and practitioner), but in my career I have learned that much more of the responsibility is on the client. In a successful case, I would say the results are 75% client and 25% our work or other outside help. Clients have to be responsible with their bodies. Health is a two-way street, and we can take them only so far. So many people reverse the percentages and depend too heavily on 75% outside help (whether through medication, doctors, etc.), and they're only comfortable with maintaining 25% or less responsibility for their own health.

When practitioners help injured bodies get back into balance, that 75% responsibility for your own health comes into full effect. But the body helps you take on that responsibility. I've seen it happen many times. After one or two visits, a client starts tapping into their own intuition about the steps they need to take to continue the healing process. For example, they start paying better attention to what their body is doing. They change their diet and stop destructive behaviors like smoking and drinking too much. They learn to recognize unhealthy emotional patterns, where they may be allowing others to step on them. The client starts paying attention to themselves for the first time in a long time as the body heals itself.

In the modern medical age, we've lost connection with the idea that the body has this capability. I'll explain this concept much more throughout the book because it is difficult to understand, but it's essential to what we do, and it will change the way you think about your own health and responsibilities.

After people ask me exactly what nerve and body restoration is, then they want to know what I do in a typical session at the clinic. I like to say that we deal with the body as a hyper-emotional, pimple-ridden teenager who just wants to be loved. When it's hurting, it needs to be cared for and know that everything will be okay. Most people can relate to that analogy. Middle school is the most traumatizing phase of life, as far as I'm concerned, and teens require a safe place to go to regroup. Usually that safe place is their home or their bedroom. That's the reasoning behind why the rooms at my clinic are not sterile treatment rooms. We designed each one with the comforts of home so that clients feel safe when they enter, which is of primary importance to healing.

We had our share of barn cats of every stripe and color on the farm growing up, and I remember hand-feeding many puny kittens with eye droppers of milk after the mother cat refused to nurse them. Mom made an exception to her "no pets in the house rule" and allowed me to keep those little guys in a laundry basket inside our home until they were healthy enough to rejoin their mother. Mom even warmed up towels in the dryer for the kittens to snuggle into and rest. It's a memory that comes to mind when I think of how important feeling safe is to healing. If we ensure people feel safe and secure with us, their body can relax much more easily. Relaxing and feeling safe allows us to get to work right away assisting a client's body out of fight or flight mode and shift it into a rest and restore mode where healing can occur.

In order to initiate the best response from our clients, we first find out where they are physically, emotionally, and mentally. We give their body enough time to slow down and be heard as the client airs their chief complaint. After I listen and understand the problem, a client will lie face down, fully clothed on a table, and I begin to explain everything that I'm going to do during the session. I keep explaining along the way, especially if I can feel or sense that someone is new to bodywork, just nervous in general, in a lot of pain, or some combination of the three.

In a typical session, the practitioner performs sequences of small stimulations, called "moves," on specific points on the body. The moves are gentle, but purposeful, and can be done through light clothing. From a biological standpoint, the moves stimulate mechanoreceptors (more commonly known as nerve endings) that are overlaid on both muscles and acupoints. In simpler language, the moves give the body a signal or message to send attention to certain areas of the body. The brain then works like a filing system to interpret that information however the body needs. It can stimulate or excite an area that needs more blood flow, for example. Or it can prompt the body to relax an area of tension.

Between each set of moves, the practitioner pauses and leaves the room for as many minutes as needed for the client's body to begin responding to the information we're feeding it. The body's response to this stimulation varies as it begins balancing the autonomic nervous system—letting the body know it's okay to relax and that there is no enemy to fight.

Sometimes the body's response is to make actual changes in the musculoskeletal system and achieve increased symmetry in a person's uneven shoulders or hips. Clients may feel the work taking place as a tap, tingle, a sense of melting or floating, or a temperature change. These effects, in turn, remove blockages to restore the normal free flow of communication in the body between nerves, muscles, etc.

"I'm going to be doing sets of moves in and around your spinal cord and in and around your body," I explain. We begin with movements at their lumbar plexus and allow a few minutes for their body to integrate those initial messages. This begins the general relaxation of the body. It's a rolling move, so I want it to result in a nice, gentle ripple effect. I want it to be like a skipping rock, not a big boulder going into the lake. "First, you will feel a rolling move," I say, "and then I'll leave the room to let that simmer. I'm not going to be gone long. I'll return in a few minutes. Do you understand?"

At times I invite the client to repeat what I just told them because I want them to comprehend what's happening and not get up and follow me out of the room when I leave! They need to know I'll be right back while the body rests and integrates the information it is receiving. Once the work has begun, we limit the talking so we can truly focus on what's happening with the client's body and "hear" with our hands.

If the moves are executed accurately, correctly, and smoothly—not in a jerky manner—the body starts to open more and be receptive. The first time I saw this phenomenon happen early on in my training, I was shocked. I stood back from the table and watched someone's muscle tissues rise and then melt open. The action is like a lotus flower on a lily pad early in the morning opening with the sun. That's what the body does on the table when a practitioner is working. By the same token, if we don't do the moves correctly, the body closes up. If we give the body sharp, jagged moves, it will close down and not do well. The move will not feel good, and the client will become anxious. Their mind will never shut off, wondering what in the world is happening. It's vital that the body trust the practitioner to receive the messages we give it.

The technique we use puts the client into a meditative state so that their subconscious can start putting everything into alignment. More on that later, but what's basically happening is that the conscious part of their awareness quiets down. It abandons fear momentarily and allows the body a much-needed chance to regroup. Many clients even go to sleep. If you remember nothing else about what my story teaches you about healing, just know that the body is extremely smart. Believe in its capability. If it's given the chance to do what it's supposed to do, then it will.

The protocols I have developed during more than 18 years of doing this work are amazingly effective. It's so encouraging to see people's bodies heal, pretty much on their own. The work is completely safe and appropriate for everyone, from newborns to the very elderly and frail. Highly trained athletes and pregnant women benefit equally, each according to their individual needs. Athletes derive enhanced performance from syncing their nervous system and other body systems to work together in harmony. Sports-related injuries also heal faster in a well-balanced body.

If practitioners are gentle, precise, and focused in every move, then the body will relax and allow us to guide it where it's supposed to go, where it wants to go. We can't tell the body how to heal or what part to heal, but we can guide it. It will do its work in its own time—when it's ready. We bring order to the body gently so the body will follow suit.

The body, however, is not naturally trusting. Most bodies are guarded because we've inherited a survival instinct. It is on edge on every front. Likewise, the mind is also generally doubtful that anything is going to work to resolve the pain. When somebody says to me, "I've come here because I have hip pain," I wait for the other shoe to drop. When it does, they add something else to the list like, "…and I've also got these other things wrong with me that you probably can't do anything about."

And I typically respond, "Try me. What else is going on?"

After I hear the other issues, I say something like, "I can't do anything about those concerns, but your body can." My job is to guide it so that it can organize itself to look and see what it can fix, because it's quite capable. Surprisingly few sessions are typically needed to alleviate the client's complaint— whether structural or functional, even if the injury is long-standing.

Believe it or not, we are made pretty well. In fact, we are fearfully and wonderfully made, just as God said. Remember that. We just have to see what each body is capable of doing, knowing that everyone has their own path in life and their own timeline to get to whatever it is they're trying to get to, especially when it comes to healing. I can't force the body to do anything. If I try to force the issue or push, it usually doesn't turn out well.

I get much better results when I coax the body along, kind of like you do when leading a horse. I didn't grow up with horses on our family's dairy farm, but one thing I do know about those guys is that if you pull or push them, they won't move at all if they don't want to. It's much better to gently direct a horse where you want it to go. The animal will come along at its own pace, as long as you're patient. It's the same way in bodywork. We meet people right where they are, and then gently guide them to wherever they need to be, the place where we, as practitioners, see that they *could* be.

The causes of pain in the body vary greatly. I can't stress enough that fear is a huge "cause" whose effect is extremely detrimental in the body. Sometimes just listening to the complaint and guiding the client's body into rest and restore mode in a session will shine a light on their real cause of pain. It will help them uncover and then deal with the root of their fear. Throughout these pages, I'll share several examples of why that's the case. I'll start with one story I'll never forget. One of my earliest bodywork experiences involved a client who told me she had insomnia. But I suspected from the start that it was related to something else entirely.

4

restoring broken bodies

DURING OUR FIRST SESSION, I asked my client to describe what was going on with her body. She stated very matter-of-factly, "I can't sleep."

I suspected there was something deeper and asked if she slept at all. As it turns out, we were eventually able to figure out her sleep patterns and determine that she was indeed sleeping, taking cat naps here and there. The problem was that she wasn't getting restful sleep and certainly not 5-8 hours of full sleep. Although she was stressed and felt like an "insomniac," that was merely a label. She was experiencing a very imbalanced circadian rhythm, an internal process that controls the sleep-wake cycle. Her doctor had diagnosed her as having insomnia, but I hoped that she wouldn't just "become" that label or cling to it as her identity.

I let her vent her frustrations during our first session. She could not hear me anyway, since her adrenals were going full force, drowning out any advice I might give her. She was in full fight or flight mode. Then I worked on her and answered her questions about the process so that we could build trust. At the second session, she was better but still maintained her deer-in-the-headlights approach to life in general. The adrenal faucet was running, but not full force like it was before. By the third session, she was much calmer. Her adrenal faucet was now merely a drip, so I took the opportunity to point out something to her. I explained how, in my experience, fear is almost always the root of insomnia.

"So," I told her, "once we know what the root cause of the fear is, we can determine what triggered that root to grow in the first place." Once that key piece of information comes to the forefront, I explained, the body will deal with it almost instantaneously. The body knows what to do most of the time, and we don't give it its due.

Humans are more comfortable slapping labels onto health conditions. The flaw in this process is that it doesn't work completely and avoids dealing directly with the issue. The labeling strategy doesn't make sense to me. I don't like to label anyone with anything for any reason. It's possible (and much more helpful) to teach my practitioners to instead identify what they are seeing in a particular case, show them *why* they're seeing it manifest itself that way, and then instruct them on what moves to do around the nerve plexuses in order to help.

All without labeling.

I never told my client she was an insomniac. That was *her* word to describe her condition. Why would I also put that label on her when she had already latched onto the diagnosis? But I did wonder why she had so easily believed what she was told. Labels wear out after a while because they are used so often as a crutch. I find it's better to deal with presenting issues one by one and go from there. The picture that comes to mind is slicing mold off a block of cheese until all that's left is a normal block of cheese.

My client took to heart what I said about fear being the root of insomnia. So what was the root cause of her fear? She had to think only a moment before she could identify an incident that had happened years before when she was a young woman. She started to tell me about it, but I stopped her mid-sentence. I didn't have to hear the details of what had occurred; her body had heard her. And now the healing would begin. The next time I saw her, she reported that she had slept soundly through the night.

It's important to pay attention to how the body is manifesting its hurdles and then proceed to take down one obstacle at a time. Sometimes it's quick and easy to clear the way, and at other times not so much. We are all made so uniquely, which keeps me fascinated with my work.

Another client was paralyzed with fear the first time she came to the clinic complaining of sciatica. She had never had bodywork before, but she was in enough pain to try it. Her fear that bodywork might make things worse, instead of better, exacerbated her sciatica. I understand that anxiety—again, it's why I work very hard to help my clients feel they are in a safe environment when they come to us. When we finished her first session, I asked her to pay attention to what was going on in her body the next few days because the positive effects of bodywork continue to play out long after the session is over.

She had a puzzled look on her face, and she asked what she should be "feeling" for.

I smiled and told her, "I don't know. But you tell me what you experience when you come back for your session next week."

I could anticipate what she would be feeling as her body began to heal because I've worked on so many cases of sciatica with positive results. But I didn't want to predict anything for her. I avoid putting thoughts in my clients' heads because that is a way of leading them down *my* path, and that's not fair to the body. I couldn't tell her what her unique body would be feeling.

The work we do typically extends the healing process for a period of five days after a session. The nervous system, for example, takes an average of five days to repair itself and make changes. The client will usually feel most of the expected sensations within the first 36 hours after the session. Then they dissipate and are not as "loud" in the body.

If the body can jump to it and get busy healing, it will take care of what is wrong in short order. The next week, the client told me in perfect detail about the healing sensations and tingles she had felt in her leg since I'd seen her. The body did just what I needed it to do.

"You knew that would happen, and you didn't tell me,"

she mused, still amazed at the progress she'd made in just seven days.

I explained that her body was way smarter than I was, and we were going to trust it. "It knows you, and it knows what to do for you. I am just the facilitator," I assured her.

Another lady came to see me with pain in her foot, although she didn't know what she had done to cause the injury. She told me she got up that morning and was standing in the kitchen making coffee when she felt something "slide" inside her foot. Then her foot swelled to the point that she had trouble bending it. I worked from her knee to her foot and determined that it felt as if a tendon had slipped out of its groove. I performed a few moves, left the room, and then by the time I came back inside, the swelling was already going down.

She remarked how she could "feel" her foot healing and described it as something "running around in there"—circling and swooping from her toes throughout her foot. That's the electrical nature of this type of bodywork. Medical science describes the nervous system as a series of electrical synapses. In the simplest terms, a synapse fires and sends a spark that the brain captures. It sends the information to the right factory in the body to deal with whatever organ or tissue is in distress. Some clients describe feeling a current—an electrical "zing"—that works its way from the neck to the fingers and toes. That description makes sense. You are connected from head to toe, aren't you? It's similar to the feeling you have when you hit your funny bone, which has an uncanny resemblance to being shocked (if you've ever had the unfortunate experience of touching a live light socket!).

We are all more sensitive to energy than we realize. There is an electromagnetic field around the Earth and around each one of us, which is one reason why our bodies are susceptible to the effects of solar flares. We are also 80% water, and electricity and water have a powerful reaction when they encounter each other. When I am working on someone, I can feel the sensation of energy running just under the surface. It's like the hum of an old-fashioned Edison bulb. As the session goes along, that electromagnetic field expands and keeps expanding, reorganizing as the body heals. Practitioners can feel this energy when they walk into the room with a client; it feels like walking into a cobweb. The cobweb can be cool or hot, thick or thin, depending on what is going on with a specific body. Skilled practitioners learn to sense, for example, if someone is on full tilt when they arrive at the clinic. We can *feel* a person's agitation, and that stress acts as a conductor, heating up the room. Halfway through a session, the client's body typically begins gelling or melting into the table. Instead of the muscles being firm and taut, they are now softening, opening, and flattening as the body begins to cool.

Part of this biological response is also a sign that the body is reducing the inflammation, which most of us carry to certain degrees. The body knows how to put on its own ice packs to cool off and syphon away inflammation as the electromagnetic field shrinks. By the time the client turns over onto their back for the remainder of the session, their electromagnetic field is significantly smaller, just hovering around them. The room feels quite cool, and clients often request a blanket at this point.

As I continued to work on this particular client with the foot injury, she made an astute observation and asked if there was a connection from her foot to the right side of her nose! There are actual nerve endings near your toes that control the sinuses. She said, "I can feel this in my nose, and then it goes back down to my toes." After 15 minutes of work, she stood up and declared that her foot was completely better. And it was.

The other route she could have taken is the more traditional one involving X-rays (which would have showed nothing). She may have ended up wearing a clunky boot for several weeks. In our clinic, it took about four moves in one session, and then I let the body do the rest. I'm telling you, the body is way smarter than we are. I'm just the button pusher.

One of the most helpful realizations I made early on in my career is that some people do not want to get well. It sounds counter-intuitive, but it's true. I once worked with a client who got up and left unexpectedly in the middle of her second session. I was confused and assumed that she had suddenly become ill or, worst case, had had a terrible experience somehow.

What I learned later was surprising. She told me she had progressed a lot since her first session and could "feel" she was getting even better while she was on the table in the second session. But, she admitted, she didn't really *want* to get better. Everyone in her life had accommodated her illness for so long, babying her and doing everything for her, and frankly she was not ready to give that up.

"I thought you wanted to get better," I inquired.

"I did and I didn't. I actually didn't think you could help me," she confessed. This client has since brought me many referrals, but I remember her story because of what it taught me about human nature and healing.

I have a unique take on what it means to be healed. Healing, to me, means being content in every aspect of your life. If you can feel contentment through your surroundings and in your circumstances, you will also start to feel it on the inside. When your body is telling you there's something wrong, it will start to throw up little red flags. You don't feel quite right on the inside. There is something gnawing at you. You wouldn't necessarily know that "this" ligament or "that" tendon is off kilter. You just know that something is not right with your body. Pay attention to what you are feeling. So many people do not pay attention—they just go about the motions of the day and ignore their body. I've learned not to ask people, "How are you doing?" because they usually say "fine" even though we know that's not true, or they wouldn't be there in the clinic. I've learned instead to ask people, "How is your *body* doing?" That provides a better answer.

Until you slow down and allow the body to show you the piece of your life that needs to be addressed, you will be off-tilt and discontent. We can fix the physical issues in our clinic, but those aren't really the crux of the matter. My observations and experience show me that when someone is emotionally healthy, and immersed in contentment, that person very rarely experiences injury. The body runs properly when it doesn't have to worry about emotional issues constantly gnawing at it. Once you feel that full sense of contentment, I think that is when you're "healed."

Sciatica is a popular complaint in my clinic. Your sciatic nerve is as big as your pinky, and it is an emotionally-triggered nerve. It stems from the lower back, which is your body's foundation, and controls the motion of your legs. If there is something bugging you emotionally and you feel as if your foundation is being rocked (but you're somehow holding it together), as soon as that issue is over, then your low back "foundation" cracks. It's like a little earthquake. And guess what ? Here comes sciatica. I've seen it over and over throughout my years of doing bodywork.

Clients come in to see us and say that they have "bad sciatica."

"Did you fall?" I want to know right away.

"No, I just woke up with it," comes the all-too-common response.

"Okay, then tell me about the three to six months prior to this happening," I suggest. I want to know in a nutshell if there is something more stressful that's been happening behind the scenes. Very rarely will sciatica come on without a negative emotion attached to it. (Unless someone has been injured in a fall or some sort of accident.) It is usually caused by a negative emotion or negative situation that a person has been dealing with for three to six months prior to pain showing up in the body.

"No, I can't think of anything," again comes the common response.

That's okay because if we leave the issue alone and begin working on the client, a revelation usually makes itself known halfway through the session. We're not usually talking during sessions, and we typically work in silence. However, clients often have a need to break the silence. And when they do, it turns out there has been a death in the family. There was a financial crisis. Something changed at work. Aha! Now we're talking. (Rather, they are talking and I'm listening!)

When my daughter was two years old, my mother-in-law gave some great advice about listening. She said to me, "Learn the word 'oh' in every octave. You'll understand why later, but learning to say that will keep a lot of fuel from being dumped on the fire." I learned the benefit of that technique in short order as a parent. Let's say a teenager wants to stay out way past curfew on a school night. Instead of combating and yelling, "What on earth are you thinking?" that's your opportunity to practice this technique and say in various octaves, "Oh? Ohhhhh. Oh!" And so on. It turns the volume down and avoids confrontation so you can talk rationally about the situation.

I use my mother-in-law's advice in my clinic more than I ever did with my own child. I listen as clients self-discover the root cause of their pain—avoiding any confrontation or leading from me. People like to be guided, but that doesn't mean they want unsolicited advice. They often don't let advice soak in unless they ask for it anyway. Instead of wasting a lot of breath, practicing saying "oh" in every octave simply acknowledges they've been heard. It validates the body's experience of pain. I hear, but I don't necessarily have to respond because *they hear themselves,* and suddenly it's clear what caused their pain.

Back to the sciatica example. I don't make the immediate connection for them between the crisis event and sciatica. Again, that's not my job. After I've practiced "oh" in every octave, I usually offer something benign like, "Well, that's a stressful situation. And just so you know, the sciatic nerve responds to heavy emotion."

I typically see more male clients complaining of sciatica in the spring, the same time as wedding season. Let's say the dad doesn't particularly like the guy his daughter is marrying. He goes through the motions of the wedding planning, dress rehearsals, and the wedding day because that's what's expected. After it's over, the low back pain starts, and sciatica shows up like clockwork. He tells me he's had back pain for three months, the same number of months since his daughter married the guy he can't stand.

There is a very significant pattern to this problem. I could pull hundreds of files to prove it. When the client and I discuss the trigger issue in casual story-form in conversation, it brings the problem front and center. It's no longer buried. Once this reluctant father of the bride brings his trigger issue to the surface, the body will automatically deal with it. The subconscious will raise whatever the issue is, siphoning it up from the bottom where he's stuffed it so the body can address it.

The nervous system identifies it, and this is the mysterious part, the body says, "You know what? This is going to be okay."

The father doesn't need to rehash the issue with me. The body immediately knows what's going on, and the body goes to work. Our work merely compartmentalizes and corrects the situation in the body. The sympathetic and parasympathetic balance out, and the client will reframe the pain and usually say something like, "Oh, is that all it is?" If we know the trigger, the body can deal with it. It just needs a few buttons pushed here and there when it is discombobulated.

If you find yourself in a whirlwind of stress, think about what your trigger is. Name it. Find that trigger. The insomniac found hers. The father of the bride found his. It all circles back to that issue.

Early in my career, I flew to Michigan to help another Bowen instructor. One of the clients I worked on there was a woman with infertility issues. This was a first for me, but I did my best with her. At the end of the session, she told me that she had given birth to a stillborn child in the eighth month of her last pregnancy.

Then she went on to describe to me several visions, for lack of a better word, that she'd had while I worked on her. While she was on the table, it was as if a reel from a movie projector popped into her brain. She could see her failed pregnancy happening on the screen. Then someone threw out that movie reel, loaded another, and the next scene showed up on the screen. In this scene, she described something like a giant ice cream scoop appearing to scoop out all the "bad" that was in her gut. The client wasn't afraid of what was happening. In fact, she was completely unemotional talking to me about it, but she admitted that she had quietly teared up while she was on the table watching these scenes play out in her mind.

At the end of the session, she remarked how stable she felt, saying it was the first time she'd felt like that since the miscarriage more than four years prior. I later learned that she was able to get pregnant again and carried the baby to term. Her story is simply a reminder to me that we are facilitators to help guide people into a healing state—the body does the rest.

Our subconscious does strange things. You may have learned in seventh-grade biology that REM is the deep sleep phase when the body does most of its repair work at night. My practitioners coax bodies into a REM state and ultimately to a Theta state (producing specific brain waves while sleeping or dreaming) to stimulate the body to begin healing. My guess is that this experience of total relaxation allowed this client's mind to wander freely through several images that she interpreted as movies being shown on a screen.

Body and nerve restoration pulls even the most Type-A personalities out of ego, a psychological term for the natural self-centeredness that comes hand-in-hand with human. So when the client is in that REM/Theta state, it allows the subconscious more freedom to do its job. It moves the conscious selfishness (that we all have) out of the way. When a client gets up from the table after resting in REM/Theta state, the effect is dramatic. They often even look like a different person! It affects their entire body and personality.

They come in stressed to the max, but when they leave, their brow is no longer wrinkled and their mouth is not bent into a scowl.

When people are in pain, or their lives are falling apart, they get so self-absorbed that sometimes they are their own worst enemies. And when they are so self-focused, they make bad decisions. For example, they often lash out at others. Anger and resentment are right at the surface, and it takes very little to set someone off. Clients also tend to stuff their bodies full of everything that someone suggests might help them. They are desperate and start buying every vitamin and herb off the shelf, which is not the best idea because natural remedies can be just as bad as mixing medications. More on that later.

I tell my practitioners to view clients as "packages" that come their way. And they are to do the best job they can. If the package is torn to shreds, like we've all seen in our mailboxes from time to time, it requires a different approach. You must be more fine-tuned and focused on how you are going to help that body, that "package." We work on bodies, not personalities. But sometimes the bodies are exceptionally difficult to deal with if the practitioner allows a client's negative personality to affect them. The most difficult client is the driven man or woman who hates to sit still in the clinic. They could care less about what their bodies are going through—until they can't go anymore. These personality types tend to go on full throttle until they crash. Then they want to be fixed, right then and there! It's going to take a little more time with that type of personality. Healing is not going to happen overnight.

We try to set the personality aside. I have learned to compartmentalize the body and the personality, and I coach my practitioners to do the same. That said, if a client has a poor personality, it is harder to help them. If we can set emotions aside and look at their body as a package that we're taping back together, it's a little easier.

Personalities can also change because of effective bodywork. When clients feel better and pay less attention to their own problem, they give more attention to others. Instead of being self-absorbed with their pain and concerns, they start noticing what's going on around them and treating others with more kindness. Their personality becomes whole again. Instead of this nasty, distraught, torn-apart person, they become softer.

The connection between our focus and our health is undeniable. Some people are so wound up inside of themselves that it leads to chronic pain. Life is all about their fragile ego or the fact that they are not getting the attention they need from something or someone. When they're self-focused, their body suffers. Sometimes the best (and cheapest) remedy I can recommend is to get outside of themselves and do a lot of volunteer work. Seriously. They get away from their own self-analysis, and suddenly they feel better. I suggest that some clients volunteer with animals, children, or senior adults—anything to take their focus off themselves. As they focus less on self, the body balances out and the healthier they remain.

There are clients who are extremely emotionally distraught because everything hurts. I've had people come into the clinic who take their pain out on my front desk staff. I remember a woman whose hormones were so out of balance that she couldn't see anything or anyone beyond her own pain. Everyone around her received the brunt of her negative personality because she couldn't see past herself and her own issues. The receptionist put her in a treatment room and wished me luck.

I walked in, and she began vomiting negativity with her words. And it wasn't just about her pain; it was about everything that was bothering her. She was coming apart at the seams mentally, emotionally, physically, spiritually—everything was completely falling apart. As difficult as it was to listen, I gave her the safe space to vent. I'm not a counselor by any means, but after doing a few moves and mainly just listening to her, she was a completely different human being at the end of our session.

Ironically, when a client is emotionally torn to shreds, we actually do less work. We do a little bit at a time, let the glue set, and see if it holds. In the next session, we can do some more and let that glue set. If we encounter someone torn to shreds emotionally, we say that body or that package is in trauma. By doing less to it in terms of moves, the body doesn't have to work so hard to pull itself out of trauma. It does the work bit by bit until it's healed. Soon the package is back together and beautiful again.

This angry hormonal client didn't *look* the same at the end of our session—she was relaxed and even had a faint smile on her face. Sometimes people just need a sounding board, and then everything falls back into place. The moves took her body out of trauma and put it into a rest and restore state.

Before she left, the client apologized to my receptionist and described feeling as if she'd had no control over herself and couldn't stop her rage. When she got off the table, she could resume full control of her emotions again.

Pain leads to self-absorption, and selfishness makes it difficult for us to see past ourselves. The body is sending up flares—"Help me! Help me!" That's where this work comes in. It is a privilege and quite fascinating to intervene.

It's not just a job. You don't want to take it home at night, but that's almost impossible to do. A practitioner in my line of work must *want* to help people, and you may not make much money. One person could require three hours of work in a single session. But it's worth it in the end. There's a different kind of rewarding pay off, and I'm constantly re-investing myself in the business so that we can help even more people.

I do what I am *called* to do—and if you're lucky enough to love what you do for a living, you know what I'm talking about. I don't consider it a sacrifice. Just as soon as I think about cutting back my hours at the clinic to focus on other aspects of the work, I meet someone like Robb. Over four years ago, he came into our clinic. I wasn't sure I could help him. I only knew immediately that this client would take much more time and focus than I'd ever given to that point in my career. But what I *didn't* know was how much he would change my life.

5

one man's story
changes everything

A friend of mine was receiving treatment from Lynell
for headaches and back problems for some time. He
kept telling me about her clinic and suggested I go
see her. He told Lynell about me and the severity of
my injury to see if she was even willing to see me.
When my friend told me that Lynell had agreed to give
it a shot, I made an appointment in January of 2017
at the start of my eleventh year since the accident.

—ROBB, 2021

ROBB'S LIFE CHANGED one weekend in 2005 on what was supposed to be a fun guy's trip right before Christmas. They arrived Saturday night and planned to stay until Wednesday, spending all their waking hours riding four-wheelers in the sand dunes around Yuma, Arizona. Robb, a very experienced dirt bike rider, intended to bring his bike, but his truck had been so full of camping gear that a friend had volunteered to bring it for him later in the trip. In the meantime, Robb borrowed his wife's four-wheeler for the dunes. On Sunday morning, he and his friends got up early and went for a ride. After about two hours, they decided to return to their camp.

Robb was not riding very fast when he came up over the top of a dune and hit a bush protruding from the sand. The sturdy branches hit the tire and caused the four-wheeler to stop abruptly, throwing him over the handlebars. Somersaulting helplessly through the air, Robb's head struck the sand. The visor on his helmet buried into the sand like a shovel, holding his head still as his legs bent awkwardly over his back like a scorpion tail.

Face full of sand, Robb never lost consciousness. He flipped over onto his back and tried to get up but couldn't. Reaching down he touched his legs and instantly knew he had been paralyzed. One of his friends rushed over and asked if Robb was okay.

"No, I'm done," Robb told him.

He gingerly pulled off Robb's helmet, allowing him to clear out some of the sand from his mouth so he could breathe better. Two others drove off on their four-wheelers to get help. To make him more comfortable, another friend offered to take off Robb's boots. Robb thought that was a good idea but wondered after a few minutes why his friend hadn't taken them off his feet.

"Hey, are you going to pull off my boots?" Robb asked, unable to look down at his feet.

But his friend had already pulled off the boots, and

Robb never felt a thing. Robb laid there on the sand dune for almost two hours waiting for an emergency crew to arrive in a dune buggy called a medical sand rail loaded with emergency equipment. When they finally arrived, medics loaded Robb onto a gurney and drove him in the sand rail to a waiting ambulance.

Once inside the ambulance, emergency personnel performed an initial assessment on the way to meet a med-evac helicopter that would take Robb to a medical center in Yuma. Unsure of the extent of his injury, Robb told his friends not to call his wife, Lisa, until he had more information. At the hospital, doctors examined him. Robb still has the ink spot from the pen the Yuma doctor used on his arch to see if he could feel anything. He could not. It was quickly determined they needed to send Robb to Barrows Hospital in Phoenix to see a specialist.

In a weird twist of fate, Robb's emergency flight to Barrows was delayed over three hours because an armed man had come into the Yuma ER in the meantime, threatening to shoot someone. During the delay, someone called his wife and told her the terrible news. After the hospital lifted the lockdown, the helicopter left with Robb on the way to Barrows where Lisa would be waiting.

When the next helicopter landed at Barrows and unloaded the gurney, Lisa assumed it was Robb and yelled out, "I love you!" as the nurses steered him toward the elevator. One of the nurses leaned down and told him, "Your wife is here."

"I love you too," he told Lisa when they met. "But I'm not married!"

It was another patient, not Robb, on the gurney! For an instant, Lisa felt a smile come across her lips as she realized what had happened, but it would be a long time before that smile returned.

When Robb finally did land on the hospital rooftop in Phoenix, medical staff prepared him for emergency surgery after confirming Robb had broken his back in the T7 area and also his neck at C6, leaving him without feeling from the nipple line down. Not fully realizing the severity of his injury, Robb told the surgeon, "Do the best you can. I'm a police officer, and I must be back at work Thursday. I hope you can do some miracles."

Motorcycles had always been a passion of Robb's since he was a teenager. As a young adult he became a professional road racer. He survived two terrible accidents, including a crash at Daytona while going 155 mph that somehow left him with only a raspberry on his elbow. He'd been lucky so far, but Robb was haunted by the thought that if he continued much longer in professional racing, there was a good chance he would end up paralyzed or worse.

Alongside his love for motorcycles was his dream of becoming a police officer. So when he retired from road racing, Robb decided to pursue a career in law enforcement in Arizona and enrolled in NARTA (Northern Arizona Regional Training Academy). Robb graduated at the top of his class and earned three of the top four awards, including being named Honor Recruit and scoring the highest in shooting and academics. He placed second in physical fitness. Robb continued road racing while he was undergoing the final months of training and planned to transition out of racing entirely once he formally joined the Prescott Police Department. A few months before officially entering the police academy, Robb broke his collar bone in a motorcycle crash. A compound fracture left the bone protruding through the skin, which eventually led to an infection.

After surgery and some carefully placed rods and plate, Robb successfully began the police academy training. On day one, he was ordered to perform push-ups. Never one to draw back from a challenge, Robb instantly dropped to the ground and began doing push-ups, all the while waiting to hear a "crack" when his collar bone snapped. But it held strong, and Robb soon graduated from the police academy. He became a patrol officer for the Prescott Police Department where he continued to court danger and more close calls, including a few assailants who shot at him!

When Robb broke his back on the four-wheeler in December 2005, he knew it was bad. But something told him he would probably just get lucky again, like he always had. He'd led a charmed life and truly believed he would go back to work at the police department after Christmas. In reality, he had no idea about what was ahead.

After spinal surgery at Barrows, Robb woke up several hours later surrounded by numerous friends and family members. He remained in the ICU for two weeks. Robb and his family spent Christmas in the hospital, and he began rehab. Robb's doctor had said the best chance of healing would occur within the first year of an injury like his. So Robb dedicated himself to his recovery, promising to eat clean and quit alcohol of any kind. He pushed himself in physical therapy, determined at every point not to let the injury keep him down. He even volunteered to carry an Olympic torch in a local race for law enforcement about five months after the accident. With the torch strapped to the back of his wheelchair, Robb rolled over eight miles from the local airport to downtown Prescott to help raise funds for the Special Olympics. He refused to let his situation taint any part of his life.

Fortunately, he had a lot of support from his wife and their three children, who were fairly young at the time. He didn't want to be a bad example to his kids, so he did everything he could to overcome his limitations. With modifications and assistance, he went mountain biking, sail boating, deep sea fishing, swimming, and even got certified as a scuba diver in 2009. Years passed. Despite his efforts and determination, Robb never regained feeling from the chest down.

When Robb came to see me the first time in January of 2017, we talked before we did anything else. I asked him about his injury, including what he could and couldn't feel. He told me he had an incomplete T7 injury to his back, which means the spinal cord was not completely severed. Robb also broke his neck at C6, but it did not result in full paralysis because his cord was still intact. Still, he had zero mobility and no sensation in his lower body. His core was essentially blubbery from lack of use, a long way from what it was prior to his injury at the height of his athleticism. Robb's arms were strong enough to wheel him around in his chair and to lift himself into his modified truck he drives using his hands. But the whole of his body was weak, and he couldn't do much of anything else. There was movement in his arms and shoulders, but not a lot. I couldn't blame him for relying completely on his wheelchair, but that sense of total dependency was one of the things I hoped would change over time.

I paid careful attention when Robb noted that he occasionally experienced spasms in his lower body, which he assumed had kept his leg muscles from totally atrophying since his accident. I filed this information in the back of my mind, and it gave me a glimmer of hope that there was something still alive in there somewhere. I had never encountered anyone in my clinic with the depth of Robb's injuries, and I honestly was not sure what I could do to help him. But I love a challenge, and I was willing to try because he was willing to try.

After the first session, Robb experienced a major sensational response throughout his body from the chest down. I did not find this out until later because he chose not to tell me at the time. However, I'd made my own quiet observations during the session. When he was lying on the table as I worked on him, I even saw his right leg kick. I said nothing.

A week later at our second session, I asked him how his week had progressed. He is not a man of many words to begin with, and he was rather ho hum in his response. I knew what I'd observed earlier, but I started to have my doubts since Robb was so reserved. The nerves and muscles in his body had been asleep—cut off completely—for years. After that second session, I was reminded of the extent of what I was dealing with. Did I think we could continue? Was it worth it? We'd agreed at the start that if after six to 10 sessions his body was unable to trigger or awaken any of these connections, we would not continue. I did not have a halo over my head the last time I looked, and I told him so. All I could do was try my best.

I was happy and relieved when after the third session he admitted to having sensations, similar to what he'd felt after the very first time I worked on him. He even told me he had "not felt anything like that before." Something was happening inside. He knew it. And I knew it. He described a tingling that began running down his legs from that first session and had continued for a few days afterwards. Now, after three sessions, he said that his sternum was sore. I nodded, recognizing this unpleasant sensation as a clue that his body was communicating to new and different parts of itself. It was as if his body was waking up after a long winter's nap.

While I was working on his toe pad during the third session, he described feeling a contraction of sorts in his abdominal muscles. One week later, something else amazing happened. Robb had regained about three inches of new feeling at his original injury site in his back. This new feeling extended around to the front of his ribcage. His abdominal muscles continued responding as they had the week before when I worked on his feet. We took all of this as another encouraging sign.

I think we were both impatient for the next week to roll around, since Robb had experienced tremendous progress in such a short time. He now described feeling some sensation at the point of his hip bones, all the way around, although it was a dull sensation. His legs at this point had become incredibly tingly, giving him the strong sense that they *could* move—a major milestone. If it were possible to "see" someone's regaining their hope...someone who had gone so long without it...I saw it that day on Robb's face. And I felt it, too.

By the end of six weeks, Robb's abdominal muscles began responding on command when I told him to practice sucking in and pressing out. He said afterwards that his torso had been very sore for three days, but it was a good kind of pain because it meant he was regaining degrees of sensation and muscle growth that had been lost.

"I like that feeling," he remarked. Most people do what they can to avoid being sore, which is why many neglect exercise. Instead, Robb welcomed the tenderness and fatigue as a sign of life returning to his body. If he felt sore, the key word was that he "felt" anything at all after over a decade of having no feeling whatsoever.

After six weeks, he also experienced an intense tingling down both legs and could identify pressure and sensation from his injury site down to his hip bones. Something new was happening on another level. He could now hold in his abs, sucking air in and holding it for a few seconds. Some feeling had also returned to his right glute. With assistance, he managed to sit up straight and maintain his posture. Having a strong core is so important to the proper functioning of the human body, and I was particularly pleased to see his core tighten so quickly.

By eight weeks, he made his own discovery of how well he was doing when he was sitting in his shower chair at home and dropped his washcloth. Without thinking, he bent over to pick it up and sat back up. That's when he realized he had not bothered to strap himself into his chair like usual. He yelled for Lisa. "Come and see this!" He was excited to show her he was sitting upright in a wet shower chair without help.

When Robb came to me at 42 years of age, I started working at the core because that's how I was trained. We begin work at the point where life began, at the umbilical cord, and work outward from there. Tom Bowen said to take the body back to its origination. Core strength is something we continually work on, even today many years after we first began working with Robb. I often have him place his fingers to feel his stomach muscles tightening as they should, sending a message to his body and brain that feeling is slowly returning to that area since his injury at age 31. As we got to know each other better, and he became a familiar face in our clinic, we joked with him that he used to have a jelly belly. And now, he doesn't. The body typically puts on a protective layer of fat after an injury. Consequently, people also gain weight when they feel an emotional need to protect themselves. When Robb began to work his core, he lost the flab. He eventually got so strong in his core that one-and-a-half years later in the fall of 2018, Robb went to a water sport function put on by Barrows Neurological Center for paralyzed people. His wife videoed him water skiing while seated on a modified single ski—without being strapped on it!

When we first began, it took two of us in the clinic to lift Robb up onto the table so I could work on him. He could get up there using the strength of his arms, but two practitioners had to manipulate his lower body weight to position him where we needed him. It was difficult work to hoist him onto the table, but we did it. After four months, however, I decided that I wasn't going to do that for him anymore. It may sound like tough love, but I told him he would have to figure out how to get himself on the table for our sessions. When I issued that challenge, I knew he had the physical strength to succeed. I understood that his core had improved enough to do it—but like anything else, Robb needed to try it to prove it to himself. And you know what? He figured it out. He was able to get himself on the table in the right position while I held his legs for stability.

A significant benchmark came six months into our work when he was able to do a push up on the table. The following week he tried performing what's called a cat/cow position in yoga where you arch your back (cat) and then sink your spine (cow). His whole lower body began sliding right off the table the first time he tried. We both laughed at this near-miss, and he immediately wanted to try it again. This time I held his feet, and he was able to complete the movement.

Robb just kept getting stronger and stronger, and I was constantly thinking of various exercises for him. First, I had to demonstrate how to do it, and then we would break it down into multiple steps how to accomplish it. Once I demonstrated how to do a new exercise, he didn't forget it, but he had to *learn* or re-learn how to do it. Because he hadn't done these movements in so long, his brain needed more time to recall all the steps involved in completing the action. I could tell you to get on all fours and perform a cat/cow, and you'd know what that was and how to do it. But Robb's brain didn't know that.

I also had to teach him how to roll over from his back to his stomach and vice versa in a better, healthier way. He had long been treating his non-functioning legs like two sacks of flour, using momentum from his upper body to get his legs to come with him whenever he turned over! Or he would grab his legs with his arms and just throw them over. It was painful to watch, as if his legs didn't belong to the rest of his body.

I feared he would injure himself sooner or later and explained that he could not continue to do that. Robb had to take control of his lower body and roll over, as if his legs were attached to him, despite the fact that he could not feel them. To demonstrate what I wanted him to do when he rolled over, I had to lie on my back and ask myself what steps were involved in turning over. I practiced these individual steps so that I could break it down and tell him how to do it step by step. He asked me to show him again and again, and then he gave it a try. It took some practice and a lot more effort to turn and bring his legs with him in a slow, deliberate manner. But he did it.

Robb learned these new skills about nine months into our work, the same time when he learned to sit up straight, without help, on the edge of a chair.

"Look at this!" he said one day, grinning, as he sat up unassisted for the first time. When his upper body eventually collapsed into his hips, he was even able to suck in his belly and return to a sitting position.

"Good, that's your homework exercise," I informed him. When he was at home, I added, he couldn't be in his wheelchair. I challenged him to sit on the edge of another chair or the couch and use his core muscles to hold himself up, recovering again whenever his upper body collapsed. His back cramped when he tried it that first week, but it would get stronger in time.

"Don't be lazy," I encouraged. The wheelchair was making and keeping him lazy, and he knew it. Those wheels had substituted for his legs long enough.

A pattern soon began to emerge where Robb would regain some level of feeling and sensation in three-inch increments. Three inches! The progress was staggering. Not only that, but everything, from his strength level to muscle tissue, seemed to follow three- to four-month increments of improvement. I don't really know why. But it makes sense. The body's sensory cells turn over about every three months, which corresponded with the changes I observed that first year and in the years after that.

At the same time, part of the pattern was discouraging because it also included plateaus after about three months of progress. When he hit a plateau, nothing appeared to be happening. And nothing seemed to be getting better. Robb is a high-achiever, and this temporary delay frustrated him, especially since he started hitting the plateaus just as I was pushing his body more and more. Patience became the name of the game. I had a suspicion that his body was simply taking some time to heal on the inside. Just because we couldn't see any outward progress didn't mean he wasn't continuing to move forward deep inside on a cellular level. But it was hard to put on the brakes and wait for the body to catch up.

The plateaus were also emotional struggles. Robb would start to doubt and complain and even get angry at himself (which isn't like him) because he wasn't progressing like he had been. I like to say he would get "fussy" during these plateaus. All this frustration was a signal to me that whatever was transforming on the inside behind the curtain was about to become known to us in a real, observable way somewhere in his body. Sure enough, after about three months of plateau, his muscles would change, reconfigure, and grow, producing another level of soreness and achiness.

When Robb went through a serious flu-like illness, we knew his body was harboring something unusual. I learned from Robb that when you're in a wheelchair and you have a catheter all the time, you always have a low-grade infection. The body gets used to functioning in that state, but this time he was hospitalized with a very high temperature. I paid attention to the fact that it happened during one of his plateaus and that no one else in his household became ill. Looking back, Robb and I think this episode was yet another reminder that the body was doing a great work inside, and this experience was just an unusually high hurdle for the body to get over. He got better, and that would prove to be the only time that this degree of illness happened.

The next year in 2018, his progress continued in three-month increments with accompanying plateaus. A significant milestone was that Robb was able to do a side bend and return to sitting upright unassisted. That task takes a lot of core strength and engages all the muscles. Prior to learning how to do this, Robb would have to employ some herky-jerky movements just to reach a slip of paper or other object that fell out of his lap when he was sitting at his desk. Then he'd have to hoist himself back up, pulling and pushing with his arms instead of his core.

After a few times of painstakingly bending his torso and collapsing, he repeated the side bend for me until something clicked finally, and he could do one without straining. The next week he could do several side bends in a row, perfectly.

The injury to his neck was slowly healing as well. The muscles had not yet re-developed there, which made it easier for me to get right to the nerve lines and feel them buzzing like an electric fence. I could actually feel the zing of his nerves, awakening and repairing themselves—picking back up where they left off years ago. It made me think of my brother and all the times he played tricks on us with the electrified cattle fence, but I was thankful at the same time and smiled. I know what progress feels like in healthy nerves. It is like a humming, which is what Robb was feeling in his legs on certain nerve lines when I touched them, like the gluteal nerve and sciatic nerve. Every time I moved over a certain nerve line, I felt the vibration in my fingertips. And his legs would move!

I had my other practitioners observe this as a learning opportunity. The average person would not know where to place their hands, and you must develop a hyper-sensitivity to feel the vibration. But they could all feel it. It was so noticeable. I was proud of my practitioners. Robb was amazed too, silently watching his legs move on their own accord when I touched his nerve lines.

I tell my clients that body and nerve restoration work allows me to "see" what their nervous system is capable of doing. That's when we get a question like, "How can you actually *feel* the nervous system?"

That's when I take a firm hold of their ulnar nerve (that runs

across your elbow/funny bone) and ask, "Can you feel that?"
That usually answers the question.

Yes, a trained practitioner can feel a lot of the nervous system. Not all the nerves, of course, because there are so many. They're like the roots of a tree with big roots and little feeders. We send messages in certain areas to prompt those feeders to send messages back to the root nerves like the sciatic, gluteal, and ulnar. We can work on a body that has been in chronic pain, then give it a week to let the body do its job. Sometimes clients say the next week that the pain went away for three days and slowly returned. That is not bad news. It's a clue that your body is capable of healing. Because if it's able to take pain away for even a moment, it means it's capable. Because of my experience with bodies, I know the pain can eventually go away completely. A client with scoliosis once told me after we worked on her, "I honestly forgot that I had back pain." The nervous system is more capable than we realize. Another client brought in a months-old baby with "bouncy eyes." They looked like basketballs dribbling in his eye sockets. A doctor had said it was a result of underdeveloped nerves and planned to do surgery on the tiny baby, the mother explained to me when she brought him to the clinic.

"Well, let's help the nerves develop," was my response. I performed a series of moves to set the foundation and stabilize his cervical nerve plexus around his head and neck. Then I moved to the optical nerves, taking 10-20 seconds of waiting time between moves. The baby blinked and then both eyes stopped bouncing immediately. This held for several weeks. When the bouncing returned, we saw him on a regular interval of sessions for a while. He is a healthy 10-year-old today—and no bouncy eyes!

I tell these stories because that's the power of the body. The next significant benchmark in Robb's story came in the fall of 2019, a few months before another game-changing event took place around Christmas. I had observed for some time that Robb's quad muscles were re-developing. How could that be? I wondered. He had not put any weight on his legs since his accident. Still, I could not stop thinking about his muscle development. Could we start to march Robb's legs in place and utilize the weight of his upright body? What would happen if we tried? Could he learn to stand up? To walk?

I finally asked Pete to come into the clinic to help me get Robb to stand up. I needed someone strong enough to be able to hold Robb's body in a bear hug because I wasn't sure Robb could stand. Robb and Pete were both such good sports as Pete reached down, lifted him up out of the chair, and Robb held onto his shoulders—all 175 pounds of him.

Another practitioner, Denise, was there to help us and she was likewise blown away when Robb announced he could feel his weight underneath him.

I instructed Denise to hold one of Robb's legs, while I held the other, and we practiced marching Robb's legs in place about 10 times.

"I can feel that motion," Robb said breathlessly.

Pete just looked over and smiled at me.

We sat Robb down again in his chair, and he described the extra-tingly sensations running up and down his legs. Robb was excited—we all were! We repeated this exercise every week for the next few months, and Robb discovered he was more sore, and even stronger, with each passing week.

Little did we know we hadn't seen anything yet. Christmas Eve was almost here, and it turned out to be the perfect time for an unexpected gift.

After Robb was initially injured and began to recover, the Prescott Police Department reassigned him to Prescott's 911 Call Center. It was a difficult transition from the street to an office. One of the things Robb loved most about being a patrol officer was being outside in the fresh air every day, meeting new people and interacting with his community. Now he was in a room 12 hours a day behind a computer screen, another huge and devastating blow. On the positive side, he still worked with the same people in the same line of work that he thrives on—dealing with emergencies and stressful situations.

He has served in dispatch for 15 years now, starting on the floor taking 911 calls and manning the radio dispatch for police. Determined to succeed, Robb eventually worked his way up and became the lead dispatcher before accepting a supervisor position at the Prescott Regional Communications Center, where he serves as manager of the Center today. Ironically, he is the one tirelessly guiding others—callers and emergency personnel—through their own extremely challenging situations every day. By helping him in our clinic, I like to think that we're also helping thousands of other people he works with in a community we both love.

On Christmas Eve 2019 Robb came in for his final session of the year and told me that he'd had a growing sense that he was going to stand up soon. He didn't know why he felt that way, but he described the intensity of this feeling as almost *needing* to do it. I worried that he might go down if he tried to stand up, and since it was just the two of us at the clinic with a scaled-down holiday staff, what would happen then? It freaked me out, to be honest.

"It's okay, Lynell," Robb said. "I've been on the floor many times. I can get myself up."

That's all I needed. I said, "Okay then, tonight's the night. I'm game. Let's do it."

I got a walker and brought it to him, positioning it in front of where he was sitting on the edge of the table, where he'd been every week during our session for the past three years. But this was unlike any other session. Truth be told, I'd pictured this moment a dozen times when Robb would stand on his own and take his first steps. I didn't know when it would happen or how it would play out. That moment was in front of me now, and for the first time I didn't know what was ahead, and I wasn't in control.

Both of our hearts were pounding so hard that their beat was all I could hear in my head. I held onto the walker as he reached out with both hands and gripped the metal tubing with all his might. With one swift movement, Robb stood up!

He let his legs settle in for a minute, like sand flowing to the bottom of an hourglass. I asked him how he was feeling.

"It feels good," he assured me. He could feel his legs underneath him, as he had done with my husband many times before getting in and out of his wheelchair.

"Let's try to take a couple of steps," I said, moving the walker about an inch away from him.

He held onto the walker and took a single, solitary step. And another.

I paced him aloud. Left. Right. Left. Right. Summoning all my focus on the task at hand, I think I held my breath the entire time.

He moved in slow motion, gripping the walker, as I counted out one more set of left and right for a total of six steps.

And then it hit us. How was he going to get back? I didn't know how to turn him around! Robb said to let him take six steps backwards to get back to the table. It took a good 15 minutes to complete those 12 steps, but in another way this event had a timeless quality to it, like most Christmas Eves seem to have. The experience was overwhelmingly emotional, although neither of us cried.

As I counted the six steps backwards, left-right-left-right, Robb moved in slow motion back to the table. He sat down and had a huge smile on his face—a combination of happiness and shock. We gave each other a high-five, and then I worked on him to finish the session, but my mind was a thousand miles away.

I don't remember driving home to my family that night. I think I stayed in shock for about three days. If God himself had said to Robb that night, "Be healed!" I would have dropped dead. Robb and I didn't say it to each other, but we both knew that this event marked the moment when we began to believe, "This is really going to happen." Robb was going to walk again.

6

resilience

HAVE YOU SEEN the movie *Forrest Gump*? In this movie, Tom Hanks' character wears clunky metal braces on his legs from a young age, but he can run faster than the wind. Robb received a pair of those exact type of braces from the hospital after his accident. He remembers the hospital staff telling him he would never actually *use* the braces. They had encouraged him to just "get used" to life in his wheelchair.

When he went to physical therapy the first year after his accident, he occasionally wore the leg braces because he was curious to see if they would help. The metal casing came up above his thigh and kept his legs straight, but the problem was that he had no feeling in his core and nothing to hold up his upper body. He couldn't sit up, like one of those dolls with the string in its back—you pull the ring at the end of the string and the doll comes to life briefly before collapsing. It was frustrating and not motivating.

In January of 2020, Robb and I were excited to continue practicing taking steps. But supportive braces would be essential from this point forward. It was too hard otherwise. He wore his old leg braces starting in January of 2020, and they were game changers. They were cumbersome and heavy, and he walked stiff legged, but I saw they gave him the confidence he needed to practice taking the smallest of steps. He tripled his steps from Christmas Eve by week two.

Robb did not want to invest more money in better leg braces because he, like me, had the goal of not having to use them at all. It's commonly said that the first year of physical therapy and recovery after a debilitating accident or stroke is the most imperative time in terms of your progress. Whatever mobility you have regained at the end of a year is where many experts believe you will remain the rest of your life. If you weren't on your way to achieving full recovery by one year, they say, you never would be.

I remember being told I would never walk again after my back injury. I'm not a fan of "never." It's not nice to say to someone. Especially not someone who is struggling to regain their former life before a tragedy took it all away. I am a realist, but I also want to hold out hope. When people lose hope, they deteriorate. Statistics are based on research of the masses, but our bodies are all so individual that one person can be the exception. And I'm willing to believe in that exception. I'm not interested in absolutes; I'm interested in what *your* body is capable of. I believed with all my heart that Robb would be an exception.

By August of 2020, eight months after his Christmas Eve

walk, Robb was making tremendous progress. He and I had worked on taking small steps with the walker up and down the hallway in the clinic for many months.

His body had strengthened all over by that time, and he was ready for a new challenge. We decided to go big and put him on the treadmill in September.

"We'll just give it a go and see," I told him one day.

Robb is such a willing participant. He's not afraid of anything I suggest. "Okay, let's try that," he agreed.

The way the body works is similar to the military's chain of command. The nervous system is the senior command, and it oversees all the body's activity. It tells the muscles what to do, and the muscles then relay these orders to the bones. It all works together in an orderly fashion—until there is an injury. Nothing in Robb's body was working well for 11 years because the nervous system had been asleep at its post since his accident! Challenging Robb to put in the hard work on the treadmill pushed the nerves to wake up and start regenerating and remembering all that they were supposed to do.

Robb had learned to sit and stand up by this point, and now it was time to learn to walk again. The nerves informed the muscles to come to attention—they had a big job to do, and so did Robb's bones. As the nerves regenerated, the muscles and bones fell in line and started following their orders because that is what they know how to do.

We began by putting Robb in a full bodysuit harness for his safety, and he wore his trusty leg braces. We even had a safety roll bar hanging down from the ceiling for him to hold onto if necessary. I started the treadmill at .5mph, and we took it very slowly. At first, his lower body swung wildly out of control in the harness like a marionette trying to put his legs squarely on the belt. Through tremendous concentration, Robb gained more control of his legs and hips and could place his feet firmly on the belt. Then he could take the smallest of steps. I sat behind the treadmill on the floor so I could pick up his feet one by one and plant them in the right position.

When he first began walking on the treadmill, it took everything he had within him to accomplish that task. He sweated profusely as if he were running a marathon. However, as his body got used to it, he sweated less, and his breathing became steadier. He was still putting in the work, it was just becoming easier.

I was interested in all the feedback Robb could give us about what he was experiencing. He told me it was just tingly when he walked, as if his legs were asleep, and he couldn't feel anything past that prickly sensation. It would take a long time for him to feel anything in his legs when he was in a standing position. The tingling sensation he felt was the nerves giving the muscles electrical impulses as they began knitting back together. The communication into the muscle tissue results in an intense tingle. Over time, he could feel past the tingles, and they happened less and less as more muscle tissue "turned on" while he walked on the treadmill.

After a few weeks, the chain of command was clearly working between his nervous system, muscles, and bones. His legs began developing more muscles and became heavier for me to position whenever I stretched out his muscles after a treadmill session. When he could reach down and feel with his hands how much muscle tissue was returning to his legs, it encouraged him.

He said to me one day, "When you touch my legs, I can sense there is dense tissue there, instead of just skin." That let me know he was starting to regain even more sensation in his legs. His legs had also increased circulation and, therefore, had less swelling.

One day he was being particularly fussy when he began our usual routine on the treadmill. "This doesn't feel right," he told me, pointing to his harness. (The harness was fine.) And later he complained, "I feel sore and uncomfortable. This feels weird. It feels like something's irritating me." (Nothing had changed in our set-up since the week before.) Frustrated, he completed his first round of walking.

Then I asked him to repeat what he'd been saying about all that was wrong. He looked at me funny. "Well, I feel grumpy…" he began.

"Stop right there," I interrupted. "What did you say? Pay attention to your words."

"I feel…" he began again and then the lights went on. "Oh, I can *feel* everything. That's why I'm so sore. I can feel! I can *feel*!" He could feel more muscles turning on, and they were not happy. His whole demeanor changed when he consciously connected to his words and realized what he was saying. It was a good kind of sore because it meant he was feeling something beyond just the tingles he had experienced many times. If you've never run before, and you ran a mile for the first time, you would feel your leg muscles burning the next day. Robb was at a point where he could feel more and more of that soreness. It was confirmation that his muscles were responding to nerve signals in a normal and expected manner.

From the start, I planned on taking away pieces of Robb's "security blanket" from our complicated set up on the treadmill in the back room. It was so clumsy to work with all the contraptions we had rigged up. He had a lot more crutches than he really needed, but until he felt comfortable and safe, I let him rely on as many of those as he needed.

First, I wanted to change the full body harness because I wanted him to rely on his core muscles to hold him up instead. Plus, that bulky type of harness was irritating and often got in the way of what we were doing. He also had trouble walking on the treadmill with his catheter rubbing against that bulky harness. When his core muscles strengthened even more, we eventually downgraded to a smaller rock-climbing version of a harness without the hard straps or loops he no longer needed. I tried it on first, ensuring that it was very comfortable. As a bonus, the harness also protected Robb's catheter tube without getting in the way.

Even with this change, Robb still couldn't feel enough adequate pressure or weight on his legs to simulate a natural walking stance. The core was doing its job holding him erect, but we needed more weight-bearing on the legs so that they would re-learn how to manage that weight and hold him up. We had to figure out how to support his torso, while at the same time put enough pressure on his hips and leg muscles to encourage them to become stronger like his core. When we switched to a vest-like harness for his upper body to protect him from falling, his weight rested more naturally on his legs. This change gave the proper signal to those muscles to do their job and help Robb walk.

In November of 2020, Robb stopped using the metal leg braces, even though doing so concerned him initially because he feared he could not walk without them. It was a mental roadblock, and he had reached a point where these braces were holding him back. I reminded him of that Christmas Eve moment when he had taken his first steps without any braces at all. I shared with Robb a personal story on the day he ditched his metal braces and tried on new lightweight ankle braces for the first time.

I was super pigeon-toed when I was a kid, I told him. My doctor wanted to put me in leg braces, but Dad in his wisdom suggested putting me in roller skates instead. It sounded like a good idea, but try to roller skate when you're pigeon-toed. It's hard work! After I fell a few times Dad simply said, "You'll learn."

Mom wadded up two rolls of dish towels and tied them to my knees for knee pads. Our cement basement was the perfect roller rink. I had one sister on each side of me to help wheel me around the basement so I wouldn't keep falling all the time. I started in strap-on metal skates and graduated to very cool white boot skates with purple pompoms after my legs strengthened and I was no longer pigeon-toed. Dad is the one who first taught me through this experience that the body needs to rely on itself to heal properly. Taking off Robb's leg braces would give his body the opportunity it was seeking at this point in his journey.

When Robb took his place on the treadmill to use his new lightweight braces, I sat on the floor behind the treadmill as I normally did. I remembered the days when I had to pick up his feet and place them on the belt to aid his body in the walking motion. He and I both were working very hard back then! That was history. My job had reduced to lightly tapping his heels when they got stuck on the belt. He still had a little bit of drop foot, but a small tap usually brought his heels right up and back into position.

Whispering to himself, right...left...right...left, Robb typically develops his own cadence and is lost in concentration when he's working. Athletes often go inside of themselves when they're in the zone during a workout, seeking some internal rhythm without necessarily needing verbal coaching from their trainer. Therefore, I often sit silently behind him while he is working the hardest, which is what I was doing the day he tried his new braces.

He walked 10 minutes without issues, then he rested and began a second walk. Robb was moving so well that I quit helping his heels for one minute—he was doing it all himself. He didn't know that I'd stopped helping him and continued to walk the next minute unassisted. Robb was lifting his legs so beautifully—it was shocking.

Toward the end of about 60 seconds flying solo, I let him know that he was doing it all on his own. Then he freaked out so much that his foot landed off the belt when he stepped! But he recovered, got his feet back under him, and kept going. He walked for another minute all by himself.

Feeling inspired, I got up and walked around to the front

of the treadmill. I paused the belt and instructed him to lower himself into a squat. He did so.

"Now stand up," I told him, like a drill sergeant. There was no doubt in my mind he could do it. I do have a sense of expectation when I'm working. God himself said to expect miracles. So I say, ask! What's the worst that can happen?

When I asked Robb to squat and stand up, he smirked and I assisted, but very little. He maneuvered from a squat to a stand four times. It took absolutely everything he had, but he did it. Another practitioner was there observing, along with a student I was training and my daughter who sometimes works in the office. I saw my daughter's eyes well up with tears, and she told me later, "Do you know what this is doing? It's giving him his life back." She is right.

Robb still seemed energized, so I suggested he use the walker, as I held onto it for assurance, and go from the doorway to the table inside one of our treatment rooms. There was no stopping him. He walked to the table, turned himself around, and backed up so he could sit down. This extraordinary series of moves did not tire him, and he was not breathing hard.

Most amazing of all, Robb commented that he could feel pressure in his feet on the ground as he stepped. He would later describe having very sore, crampy feet, which was entirely new territory since his feet have taken the longest to respond. That was enough miracles for one session, I assumed, so I decided to call it a day and work on him. But there was one more miracle left.

No longer carelessly flipping himself over onto his belly as he'd done in the past, Robb worked himself to his stomach on the table using great care. In doing so, his right leg fell off the edge of the table from about his knee to his foot. I said nothing, and he did not seem to notice.

We chatted about how good he felt and how well he was doing. Then I asked him if he felt both of his legs on the table.

"No, my right leg is hanging off," he conceded.

I told him to pull his leg onto the table, and he sheepishly said, "I'm not sure I know how."

Thinking rapidly about all the steps involved in this simple task, I asked him to lift his heel to the ceiling and then squeeze his legs together. "Do it like you're trying to get your right leg to meet your left."

Still lying on his stomach, he focused sharply and willed his glute to engage. His leg trembled like crazy, then it began to move. He stopped, lifted it, and moved some more—lifted and moved, lifted and moved. When his big toe got stuck on the side of the table, I pushed it lightly and he gingerly placed his leg in perfect position on the table.

"There," he said calmly and definitively, without looking behind him. "They're both on the table."

You know how your foot feels when it falls asleep? It's disconcerting when you stand up, almost as if you don't have a foot. That's what it had been like for Robb for over 10 years for his entire lower body. Only one-quarter of his body had been fully functioning since his accident, leaving three-quarters to the wind, without feeling, for over a decade. Lacking sensation and perspective with your limbs can be dangerous. Years earlier he had broken his femur after he was paralyzed when he was trying to put on his shoes in the car. He was sitting in the passenger seat and had rested his ankle on his other knee while he leaned forward to put on his shoe. But he unknowingly put so much pressure on his folded leg that it snapped. He now has a rod in that leg to add to the plate and screws from his broken collarbone. For the first time since I'd been working on him, he now had the sensation of his legs in space. That is how he knew his leg was hanging off the table. It was a major victory.

As I said, Robb is a man of few words. The past four years have shown me that he doles out few accolades and even fewer insights into exactly what he's feeling. When he opened up that afternoon, only for a moment, I knew we were on our way to even more incredible milestones in his recovery.

"You know, I have always been an independent person," he began. That was true. I had often wondered what he did with all his memories from his athletic and active past in a time when he was free to do whatever he wanted. From high-octane road racing to driving patrol cars and keeping criminals off the street as a police officer, Robb had lived fast and large in his younger years. What was it like to spend year after year trapped in a wheelchair? I could not imagine.

"I was never afraid to try new things, and it was always an adventure to me," he continued. My mind was racing, trying to figure out where he was going with this. But I stood stock still, not wanting to interrupt.

Then he did something I would not have expected in a million years. He pointed his finger toward his wheelchair and said, "That chair…" Choking up, he paused briefly and gathered his thoughts. "…that chair took a lot away from me. And I'm done with that chair."

"Yes, you are," I said, trying not to cry myself. "And away we go."

He smiled with fresh tears on his cheeks and said quietly, "Yeah. And away we go."

Robb's case is fascinating on many levels because of all that he has reminded me about the resilience of the human body. There are many movies and books about the triumph of the human spirit, but the body is just as steadfast in its refusal to give up in the face of tragedy. For example, when resuming communication between brain and body after a long absence, information is short-circuited in stops and starts at first. He had lingering tremors in his legs and a degree of spasticity as his nerves, muscles, tendons, and bones began communicating and functioning. But one thing I noticed as Robb began healing is that the longer we worked together, the more his leg muscle movements smoothed out. The more he walked and the more I worked on him, the more solid and steady these connections became.

When we began his treadmill therapy, I also noticed another insight about how long it took his body to warm up and get his stride. At every session, he walked on his toes for several minutes before his heels would drop and he could walk normally. That lag time was to be expected, and I didn't think much of it at first. It was taking less and less time for him to warm up as we made progress. But I wondered why there was a pattern to his warm up—it hovered at exactly nine minutes. His muscles would relax and give way after nine minutes and allow him to drop his heels and connect his whole foot with the belt of the treadmill.

One day I asked if, prior to his accident, Robb had typically taken time to stretch and warm up before he exercised or played sports. He said he did. When I asked him how long that usually took, his answer was not surprising: about ten minutes. Although his body has changed drastically since his accident, one thing it "remembered" doing was warming up. In an incredible example of cellular memory, Robb's body innately knows within its cellular system that it needs to warm up before being ready to go. His years of working out before he got injured had permanently informed his muscles, tendons, and nerves that it takes 10 minutes to warm up. And they comply, every time.

I continually have to think of something to challenge Robb's body and mind. I'm constantly changing up the routines and throwing curve balls at him so his body doesn't get used to anything. In 2021 I changed his therapy to include walking on his knees using a walker, which is hard for anyone to do, but much more so for someone in his condition. This took a lot of effort and intense focus, but once again he was able to do it. A few months later I introduced hiking sticks to him to use on the treadmill to practice a natural arm swing instead of holding on to the treadmill handles. I also challenged him to step off and onto the treadmill using the hiking sticks. It was very uncoordinated effort at first because it was new and extremely difficult work. Anytime I've issued a challenge, Robb has met or exceeded expectations, and much of that has to do with his positive approach to his own healing.

Robb told me one day that he always knew that God wanted him to walk again. "God just said that I'd have to wait a while for the right mechanic," he explained. As the mechanic, I run the shop the way I feel is best. For example, I do not assist Robb during a session in areas where he doesn't need my help. Everything I know he can do on his own, I make him do, and he understands that is the expectation. He just smiles and says, "I know you do it in love." I also won't let him easily make excuses or say he's "too tired" to put any more weight on his legs during a session. Since walking again is his goal, his job is to get out of that harness and not rely on it forever.

I don't let any clients rely too long on any crutch, and I am a very good breaker of habits. I usually don't do habits myself, except maybe that one cup of coffee in the morning (that I know I could take or leave). I've learned to love operating life on the fly. Growing up with a family of nine and one bathroom, we all had to adjust accordingly and roll with it every day. This spontaneous mindset affects my daily life for the better. When I run, I don't run at a certain time. I don't run every day. When I run long distances, I wear a water belt until about mile six when I get irritated with it and take it off. I hold it and run two more miles without it, and then I put it back on. Just making a small change like that can help my stride. We have to change it up, I told Robb, when he finally agreed to take the roll bar off the treadmill. He was leaning on it too much instead of putting natural pressure and weight on his legs instead.

When he tried walking the first time without the roll bar, I asked which way felt better to him afterwards. He still liked the roll bar but admitted having the harness alone was better. Satisfied with that answer, I began putting away some of the equipment to close out our session when I noticed he was working to get his legs underneath him without any prompting from me.

"Hey, check it out," he said as I looked over my shoulder at him. He was standing in the harness very straight on his own. Those are the moments we want more of.

My practitioners and I talk often about Robb's case, putting our heads together to come up with fresh ideas. One of the practitioners used to teach aerobics and personal training for new moms. She came up with the idea of having Robb walk on his knees. After he got good at that, I had him lean back on his heels and bring himself back up without using his arms. Once more, I had to show him how, and then he did it. I had him kneel and swing his hips back and forth, and he made an Elvis the Pelvis joke about being Robb the Pelvis. We have that one on video! I'm not going to lie—it was incredibly hard work, but he did it.

I remember the day I introduced him to cross body work which helps strengthen the mind-body communication. I sang him an old song I learned as a kid that has motions to go with it. We practiced "head and shoulders, knees and toes, knees and toes" reaching opposite shoulders, knees, and feet first and then working his way back up. This simple little exercise engages the left-right parts of his brain and strengthens the synapses from the body to the brain. There is a section of the brain called the corpus collosum, the highway between the two hemispheres. Working on information crossover between the hemispheres makes sure information is crossing all the way over the highway. The goal is to keep the highway full of traffic, all going in the right direction, to develop better synapses and start firing faster. The signals then get stronger as they're going throughout the body. I sped up the song to get him going pretty fast, and we cracked up because he was trying to keep his balance and do the right motions all at the same time. Who says work can't be difficult, effective, and fun all at the same time?

I found it intriguing that his brain wasn't always registering sensations by name. The overload sometimes made him feel uncomfortable because he didn't know what was happening. We used a sensory test to help his body and brain register specific sensations in his arms and legs, like teaching a child to associate objects and the names of the objects. For example, I would pinch his arm and say, "This is a pinch" and then go to his leg and say the same thing. The feeling was not as "loud" on his legs, but at least the sensations were now registering in his brain. Without a name for this action (pinch), the brain would simply feel it and say, "I don't know what this is, but it is uncomfortable." Having a label for a sensation assists the brain in recognizing it.

I have taken a straight pin and poked his upper arm and then his upper leg so that he knows it's a poke in both places.

Then I poke his forearm and his lower leg. We work from the upper arm to the upper leg because I'm assuming everything is a mirror in the body. I'm not sure if this is right or wrong, but it's working. I've also used a cold and warm spoon in the same manner as the straight pin, describing which one is which to register the feeling and action in his brain.

On his 100th session in July of 2019, while I was working on him Robb described feeling every single thing you could imagine: a burning, a poke, a pinch, a scratch, a scrape, a bruise. All these sensations were happening at one time, and it wiped him out.

"I don't know what is going on," he said, a worried look on his face. "I can feel everything, everywhere in my body."

His body and brain were desperately trying to organize a new mass of sensations returning in his cellular system. After 20 minutes of rest, he woke up feeling better. The body had done its thing and sorted through it.

I spend time researching what others do with clients like Robb. But I haven't found something that profoundly helps other than what we are already doing. I am staying open to new ideas that pop in my brain, and I'm content listening to my intuition and experience, because I see results.

Robb's body also has to work harder because it's relying on farmgirl innovations, not fancy rehab equipment and exercise machines we don't have access to. I'm a big believer in ingenuity and duct tape. When Robb could not reach the handles on the treadmill without leaning over (something I did not want him to do), I rummaged around in the clinic and found four pieces of wood that would work. I wound a whole roll of duct tape around them to make taller handles on the treadmill for him to grab onto. I knew my engineering studies would one day come in handy!

I recently worked on a client who had a stroke a year ago that weakened the right side of her body. She was devastated that she could no longer cook for her family and take care of their home, which she had been doing their whole lives. Instead of pursuing physical therapy, she wanted to return home and get back to what she knew—normal household activities like cooking meals for her kids. Instead of working out on machines, her kitchen became her gym. She retaught herself how to cook, measure, and stir with her right hand and arm.

Life gives us plenty of opportunities to return to what we normally do after illness or injury, and the body can rise to the challenge because it is more resilient than we know. I wonder sometimes if, in an attempt to rehab the body, we baby it too much. I was not raised to be babied. We are a family built on resilience. It's possible that we're doing a disservice to the body instead of helping it when we coddle it. I am adamant with my clients that they won't be babied in our clinic. I am compassionate, but when it's time to work, it's time to work.

Four years after we first began working together, in 2021 Robb now has intermittent feeling all the way to his feet. He regularly does sit ups and push-ups and has regained use of his lower back muscles. Robb can very easily lie on his back with his legs straight out, swaying his feet back and forth like windshield wipers. He can feel his legs quite clearly and continues to get aches and pains in them, similar to growing pains. The sensation comes more than it goes, but it's becoming more and more pronounced. It's just a matter of time for him to regain more feeling. For his 2020 family Christmas card, he took a picture with his wife, kids, and grandkids and was able to stand beside his wife, holding himself upright using the back of a couch. "You're so tall, Papa," one of his younger grandkids commented. I like to think he enjoyed blowing away his family and friends when they received the card in the mail!

I remind Robb and all my clients of their string of successes because it's so easy to take your progress for granted when the body starts healing itself. "Do you remember when you couldn't do this or that? And now you can?" I remind them constantly.

Reflecting is something I do on purpose, especially with Robb, because I don't want him to forget where he came from. And he does remember. He's not the average client in that respect. Many people come into my clinic with shoulder pain, we work on them, and they return the next week complaining how their knee or something else is just killing them.

"Yes, but how's your shoulder?" we ask.

"Oh, that's fine," they say nonchalantly.

People forget their successes because in the fast lane of life, they're already on to something else. People forget their challenges when they've been met, and they move on to the next complaint.

Robb has never been like that. He's always stressing

positivity, trying with all his might to go forward. But it doesn't mean that he doesn't resist something that seems scary to him. Even someone as strong and courageous as he is can balk at a challenge. One day in the spring of 2021 I told him to speed up the treadmill. He gave me a perplexed look. He had completed 173 sessions by then and had maintained beautiful and full control of his left leg for several months. I was barely helping his right leg with small heel taps as he walked on the treadmill. He was ready for some new challenge.

I didn't back off. "You're going like molasses, man," I kidded him. "So just for fun, let's speed it up!" We usually walk at 0.5 miles per hour, and I increased it to 1.0.

"Are you sure?" he asked, raising his eyebrows at me.

"No, I'm never sure about anything, but we're going to give it a go and see what happens," I replied. By making him go a little faster, he had to control more of his body more often. In the past, when his feet started to fall off the treadmill belt, he would use his upper body strength to swing his body back on. That's cheating. I cautioned him that he would not be able to do that safely at a higher speed.

"You have to practice control, and when we speed this thing up, you will *not* swing your body around. If you get off the belt, you will control yourself to get back on," I instructed him, tapping into the mind/body connection he needs to make his body and brain communicate about a new task.

It was impressive. He came off the belt only five times in 22 minutes at the higher speed. One time his leg drifted off the belt, which scared him, and he initially relied on bad habits and his instincts to flail and swing himself back into position. I was about to say something to him when I saw him close his eyes tightly and open them again. He had a steely-eyed look of determination, and I knew he was taking time to regroup. What he did next amazed me as he gently pulled his leg back onto the treadmill and kept going—smoothly and fully in control.

When he walks on his knees, it continues to be difficult because of this issue of control. Not only is your center of gravity lower when you are kneeling, your knees do nothing to balance you. The balance mechanisms are in your toes and feet. But he can't completely feel his feet right now. That's okay. Our goal is to get him stronger and build up his quads to hold and balance him instead. And it's working. It's getting better. Once his quads rebuild completely, he'll have even more control and more feeling of what's happening when he's walking—or even jogging, which is another level we incorporated in the early summer of 2021. In mid-May Robb started jogging on the treadmill, fully harnessed, and placing his feet rapidly on the belt one after another at a faster pace. He was still supported by the harness, but he could feel the pounding in his feet. Robb was unbelievably sore—and happy.

Another insight I've noticed is how well Robb responds to music when he's on the treadmill. Once he's up and walking, I put on my running playlist for him to hear. I even played the theme song from *Stripes* with Bill Murray and had him march to the beat. Music helps clear his mind so he can concentrate on what he's doing.

There's something about music and motion clearing our thoughts, at least that's the way it's always been for me and in my family. My parents were a force to be reckoned with at home, which was no surprise since they were raising so many kids. But they could also channel their farmer energy and transform into the most graceful dancing duo. They were beautiful together, gliding across the room arm in arm and taking up the entire dancefloor in elegant movements. So many of my childhood memories are of dancing with our father at weddings in our community. I remember noticing how the others in the church watched my parents dance. We weren't the only ones waiting for our turn with one of them. I remember Dad gathering us one at a time in his arms for a trip around the dancefloor. He went by age, dancing with each of my older sisters until he got to me, always the last in line. We began our earliest dance lessons with Dad by standing on his toes, and then learning to hold on tight and follow his feet with our own as we got older.

Dad could also sing and play the banjo, and Mom was the organist and choir director for our small Catholic church. All of us took turns turning the pages of her sheet music when Mom played the organ, and we all learned to sing. In fact, we *were* the choir at church, and I sang both soprano and alto. Mom expected all of us to learn to play the piano and at least one other instrument. My sister Cheryl learned every non-stringed instrument and used piano playing to de-stress herself. We sometimes purposely stressed her out at home just so that we could enjoy hearing her play! I learned the trumpet because all the other instruments had already been taken by my older brothers and sisters.

I loved to dance back then and still do. My husband

doesn't dance unless he has a few barley pops in him first, but when I hear live music, I have to get moving. And I always go for my runs with music playing in my earbuds. Music and movement smooth out the ridges and help us shake off the dust that collects in our lives. When Robb walks to music on the treadmill, it's a good distraction. In fact, dealing with distraction is another way I'm helping his brain re-learn basic skills, like how to do two things at once. I will have different practitioners pop in and ask Robb mundane questions when he's walking during a session. He's learning to focus on his answer and return to the task at hand, which is a reminder that walking and talking does not come naturally.

Uninjured people forget that most of what our body does every day is a learned skill. We learned it so long ago when we were children that we take it for granted. For example, self-control of our limbs is something uninjured people take for granted every day. Not someone like Robb. When he could feel the gurgling of his intestinal track once again, you would have thought he'd won the lottery. We also take hearing our stomach growl for granted because it's an involuntary sensation. We can't control that, and neither can he, but for years he went without feeling the gas bubbles moving through his system. He knows what it's like to feel hungry now. Hunger pains are a big deal to Robb. I didn't realize even something like that goes away with an injury like his, but he welcomed the sensation of hunger when it returned. Now he doesn't have to set a timer to remind him when to eat.

The work he is doing is extremely difficult, painstakingly correcting the mechanics of a single step. He can feel how hard it is, and he can sense the struggle and powerful efforts his lower body is making. When his toe gets caught on the belt while trying to lift his leg to take the next step, he can feel it catch. It takes a lot of effort just to correct that tiny thing. We take it all for granted as we walk around in our daily lives.

There are other signs of growth and progress as well. The less spasticity he has in his legs, the less short-circuiting of nerves. That has reduced to the point where sometimes he doesn't exhibit spasticity at all during our session. This tells me that his nerve lines are smoothing out and there's less "skipping." Imagine skipping a rock in a pond. That's spasticity. A little of it is a good thing, signaling the return of feeling. Too much of it is like a rock that skips and keeps on skipping, stirring up the whole pond.

The feet are the last parts of the body to feel consistent sensation because they are the farthest away from the spine and the injury. That will come. In fact, in May of 2021 he pushed his feet against my hands while I flexed his toes toward his nose. I could see the chain of command work its way down his body: his quad muscle engaged, then his lower leg, and then a push. The push felt like a faint touch from a butterfly wing in the left toes, but it was strong and more noticeable in the right foot. Better yet, Robb felt the push and the stretch in his heels as I bent his toes forward. His face lit up like a Christmas tree.

In the meantime, all his muscle tone is coming back as well, not just in his quads. Even though he had some muscle in his legs when we first started working together, there wasn't a lot, and the muscles that were there were extraordinarily hard. I couldn't squeeze the muscle with my hands; it felt like tissue adhered to bone. To elicit any kind of movement was not easy.

Ideally, the movements I do reach underneath the muscle tissue, tendons, and ligaments to lift them up and make room to breathe. It was very difficult to do any moves on his legs at first. His quads and calf muscles were like working a branch of a tree. Not anymore. His glutes have come back, and his quad and calf muscles are getting closer to full development, the right side more than the left. Now I can actually move the muscle tissue and tell that it's regrowing, regrouping, and softening up.

I have Robb use a measuring tape around the circumference of his legs to show him how they've grown incrementally. As the numbers increase, he can see for himself the progress he is making. "They feel like a leg should feel," he commented one day about his thighs. The first time I noticed his glutes were reshaping, I asked a few of my other practitioners to make their own observations to see if they noticed what I saw. (I'm always cross-checking myself.) I thought one of his glutes looked bigger than the other. Debbie was the first to notice the right glute developing more and looking much more round than the left. Seeing how lopsided the muscle was regrowing, we joked that Robb was half-assing it, and he laughed.

The glute muscles grew disproportionately like that for probably two or three months before the other side started regrouping. Now both sides are even, and Robb can see in a mirror that he has a tush instead a flat area. Those muscles are part of the largest muscle group in the body, and it's the glutes and hamstrings that help keep the human body erect. At the time of this writing in 2021, it might be another year before Robb is able to walk without any braces at all. The timing may be shorter or longer; I don't know exactly what the timeline will be. The main thing is that we're both confident that day will come. The body, on its own, is regrouping before our eyes and regrowing in order to strengthen itself for that day in the future.

All year in 2020 after he took his first steps Christmas Eve, I prayed that God would choose to send favor on myself and Robb and allow him to walk on this earth. And he made it so. My prayer right now in 2021 is that God will bless Robb's legs with more strength and courage to hold his body upright this year unassisted. What happens past that, only time will tell.

I understand why Robb didn't say anything to me about the sensations he experienced after the first session I worked on him all those years ago. He didn't want to get his hopes up, and I never plant a seed or a thought in someone's head. Instead, it's imperative that they discover and know for themselves that body and nerve restoration work is effective. Their bodies are fully capable of healing without my trying to convince people of that truth. I shouldn't have to convince anyone of anything.

Sometimes clients will say our clinic is their "last resort."

They have often tried "everything else," they tell me. I remember working on one guy who reminded me of John Wayne. "Well," he told me after a successful session, "I'm surprised this stuff works because my pain's been there for about 20 years." I laughed and said, "If you're alive and kicking, your body should be able to heal. You're above ground and vertical, aren't you? Then you're good."

In Robb's case, I could feel and see the trigger responses in his legs early on, long before he "felt" it himself. I could see certain muscles respond when I did movements around those nerves and specific muscle tissues. He didn't need to say anything for my benefit about it working—I already felt the twitches in his body. I could see and feel sensory movement under his skin. It was obvious he was feeling something—without his having to tell me, and I thought to myself, "Something is still alive in there." I'm always hopeful, so I just decided to plug along and see what happened. Most of the time the body wants to be well. It doesn't want to be ill, and I just help it get to a healthier place.

Prior to Robb, I worked with other clients with serious issues, from multiple sclerosis to severe neuropathy that left them unable to feel their feet or caused tremendous pain. In an impromptu study, I asked 10 of these clients to see me every week and record their progress after each session. The ones who came in wheelchairs left with walkers after 10 weeks of sessions. The ones using walking canes didn't use them anymore. One man's story was remarkable. He wanted to take his wife to Australia and drive a rental Jeep along the coast. That was his dream. But he couldn't feel his feet because of severe neuropathy, and he could not work the pedals safely. His wife drove them everywhere around Prescott. After we started working together, he came in one day to the clinic waving a set of car keys. I thought he got a new car.

"I can feel the pedals...I can feel the pedals!" he said, tears forming in his eyes. Then he handed me a gift-wrapped package and begged me to open it. He was a big Irishman who reminded me of a combination of my grandfather and Santa Claus with his white hair, beard, and boisterous laugh. Inside the box was an angel figurine. He asked me to look at what was engraved on the bottom of it. "Healing Angel," I read aloud.

"That's right. You are my healing angel," he said, beaming at me. He drove his wife all over Australia that summer, just like he dreamed.

His experience reminded me that I don't dictate the milestones of healing for a person—they do that for themselves and determine what they want to get out of each session. I am merely the facilitator to their body, to show them what their unique body is made of. I loved the angel my client gave me, but I'm no angel. The human body is the miracle worker.

7

the power of intuition

MY IRISH GRANDFATHER had a cool way of saying goodbye after a visit. He would never wave to you or say goodbye. He would roll his arms in front of him and then reel them in backwards arm over arm and that was "see you later"! His name was Owen, but everyone called him Onie. I was 22 years old when he passed. I was living and working in Grand Rapids, Michigan, when I had a dream that Grandpa was going to die.

I called in sick that morning because I had this overwhelming sense that I needed to get up to our farm. Mom wondered why I was there when I walked in our back door. She gave me a hug, poured me a glass of tea, and we sat at the kitchen table as I told her about the dream.

"Oh, for heaven's sake," she said, shaking her head at me and thinking for the umpteenth time what an overactive imagination her youngest daughter had. "He's been sleeping a lot, but you can go check on him for yourself. He's fine, Lynell."

Unconvinced, I drove to my grandfather's house. Aunt Betty, my mom's younger sister, had always lived with my grandparents to take care of them. My grandmother died many years before Grandpa did. I parked the car and let myself in the front door. Grandpa never locked his doors. No one locked their doors back then. Living way out in the country felt safe. I made my way to the kitchen, startling Aunt Betty when she saw me since she hadn't heard I was in town. I told her I came to see Grandpa, and she informed me he was resting.

"I'm sure he'll be glad to see you," she said. I nodded and went down the hall to his darkened bedroom and saw Grandpa lying in bed. He made an effort to sit up when I walked in.

Grandpa tried to smile and asked me all about my job and the rest of the family. Then he took an abrupt and deep breath. "Well, it's my time, you know," he said matter of factly. "The Lord's going to call me home today."

I didn't act surprised, because I wasn't. It's hard to rattle a Midwesterner for any reason, and this casual approach to death didn't faze either one of us. In some weird way, it felt as if I'd already lived this whole scene before, so it was not unnerving. I even joked with him and said that at 95 years of age it was about time for him to go on.

He laughed hoarsely.

"You're right. It is about damn time," he agreed, smoothing the top of the bedsheets with his wrinkled and worn palms. Then his eyes grew serious, and he told me to go get my mother. He instructed me not to return to see him the rest of the day.

I did as my grandfather told me, and Mom picked up the phone to call her brothers and sisters to come over. Grandpa died later that evening.

This was not the first time a wave of intuition washed over me, signaling what was ahead. As a child, I often anticipated that something significant was going to happen. And then, more often than not, it would come to pass and bring my vague foreboding feelings into sharp focus. It's hard to describe, this sixth sense, and I couldn't quite put my finger on it. I started experiencing this from the time I was 12 years old, and it has continued throughout my adult life, sometimes in my dreams. I don't dream often, but when I do dream there is always a reason behind them. I don't always know the reason until later, but there is a significance to those dreams. They are so detailed and real.

When we first moved to Prescott, a lady I met invited me to her Catholic church for the "blessing of the sick" service. I told her I would meet her there. I was looking for a church home, and having grown up Catholic, this type of service where they pray over people who need healing was familiar to me. I was supposed to meet her at 6:30 in the evening, but I had trouble finding the church. I stopped at a stop sign to call for directions when I looked up in the sky and saw a huge falling star trail right behind the steeple of the church! I turned and drove right into the parking lot. It seemed like it was meant to be. What I expected to happen that night and what ended up happening could not have been more opposite.

A visiting priest from Zimbabwe was leading the service. Unlike my experience at our small church in Michigan, people were lined up in the aisle waiting their turn to fall on the floor after the priest prayed over them. It was chaotic and totally strange. Part of me wanted to leave, but part of me also wanted to stay. I watched the drama taking place at the front of the church and sang along just to pass the time. I could not wait to go home.

Have you ever done something so out of character for you—but you're helpless to do anything else? Suddenly I found myself standing in line to be prayed over by the priest. Two people stood behind me to "catch" me when I fell, but I dismissed them. "Right. I think not," I told myself. "I will not be falling tonight, thank you."

The priest put his hand on my head, and then his face clouded with an almost frightening look. He backed away momentarily and said in Spanish, "Go away, Satan!" I could not move. I felt my body heat up so hot that it felt as if I were being torched from the inside out. Then just as suddenly I felt an icy cold wave wash over every part of me.

"This is weirrrrrrd," I remember telling myself. "I'm outta here." And I left. That night I had an unforgettable dream. I'm more certain of the meaning of my dream than I am of whatever happened at the church with the Zimbabwe priest.

In my dream I was in a dark forest holding on to a black piece of coal against my chest. I was trying to make my way to the edge of the forest where I saw a light shining, but something was holding on to my leg. Looking up, I saw a mammoth-sized eagle circling overhead three times and crying out in a loud screech before it dove straight toward me. It encircled me three more times, so fast that my hair was blowing. Then it stopped directly in front of me and stared at me with eyes that could melt anyone. I wanted to speak and plead my case so it would not harm me, but I had no mouth. My eyes were suddenly like movie reels playing my whole life before me. The eagle watched the scenes with great interest, occasionally looking at me as if trying to decide if I were worthy to save.

"I guess you'll do," it seemed to conclude when the movie was over.

Before I could blink, he took one of his great wings and soundly walloped whatever had been holding onto my leg. At that, I was free, but all the color went out of my dream. The eagle lifted off and circled me three times again before quickly snatching away the black lump of coal I was clutching. The lump grew larger and larger between his talons as he flew. He cried out three times, and then he was gone.

I looked at my feet and saw a river of water forming underneath them, through and under my feet. Huge, lush green plants with flowers of every color began to fill up the banks of this flowing river, and I found myself in some sort of paradise. Then I woke up.

I believe dreams can be a way of God communicating to you in a way he can't do when we're awake. When we're awake, we're busy. We may feel something nagging at us, but we don't know what to do with it until the body goes into rest and ceases its everyday worries and concerns for a few hours. Dreams carry messages—not every dream—but the clear, finely-detailed dreams like this one usually have something to tell us.

This was also the case after my brother Daryl died a few

years ago in a tragic accident at work. There were about 900 people at his funeral, so many that the church put speakers out in the parking lot for the overflow. I believe that when someone passes on, something new appears. When my niece, Daryl's daughter, got married, they had difficulty getting pregnant. After the birth of their first child, trying for a second baby was even harder. During that time, I dreamed that my brother was standing next to Mom in heaven. Mom was sitting in a rocking chair, holding a tiny baby boy.

"Tell her this little boy is for her. He's not ready to come there yet, but he'll be ready soon," Daryl said to me. In my dream, it was as if the baby was still developing in my mother's arms. The next day I called and told my niece about the dream and then forgot about it. When she became pregnant several months later, she let me know the sex of the child—a boy, just like Daryl had said. He was born in June 2021. This dream was as comforting to me as it was to my niece.

If you have a dream that seems to have meaning for you, pray about it. See what's there. Pay attention. After the whacky experience at the church and the unpredictable eagle dream that same night, I felt certain I was going down the right path in my life. The dream gave me confidence that I was worthy enough to pursue my goals of running my own business. Everything started going my way from there on out. Any obstacles were removed, and good things were ahead.

Rapidly taking in all the details within my environment came easy to me when I was young. I was a very observant child and paid close attention to undercurrents of information that most people seemed to overlook, including sensing people's moods and recognizing personality quirks and habits. In a house full of people and chaos, I did a lot of sitting back and watching as if I were looking at actors on a stage. Soft-footed, I often entered a room without anyone knowing I was there, which was fine by me because I just wanted to take my seat and see the rest of the play.

Reading people was a skill I developed early in life. Learning to scan bodies for information came later. I use this combination in my professional life by observing what's happening in my clients' world and then scanning to see how it shows up in their bodies. For example, some people are aloof and pretend not to be stressed, but their body tells me a different story. When and how I can point out that disconnect to a client is tricky, and this type of work requires an innate sense of timing. It's something I've learned over the course of almost 20 years in this field—reading people and knowing what's going on without their having to say it.

I don't know how to explain that. Intuition is a gift I didn't ask for, but I received it. It is hard to teach intuition to others, but it is possible to learn it. In this work, it helps to be observant enough to watch someone's body language and take in everything about them in a very short amount of time to know what to do to help them. I'm constantly thinking, "Yes, I can say that now." Or, "No I can't say that yet." I must sense when I can do that move or this move, or when I cannot do a move because it would be too much. I'm still working on my poker face because I haven't yet mastered that!

Sometimes when I'm working on someone I find myself so zeroed in on the destination where we're headed that I can't help thinking that maybe he or she could get there a little faster. But when I see that the client is nowhere near thinking along those same lines, I slow down and practice patience. Normally, I'm pretty even-tempered when driving in my car or standing in the grocery line. (Unless I happen to be having a hormone flash. That's a different story.) Patience pays off in a number of ways in my work, and I teach by example how to wait for the body to do its thing when it comes to healing.

In other words, I can see where a body "is" when someone is lying on the table. But I can also clearly see the ideal place where that body needs to go. That ability to visualize what needs to happen next in someone's healing journey comes from having observed thousands of bodies for so many years. Again, I don't try to push for a result, but I coax the body in the right direction.

It's observational skills, not rocket science. When someone is complaining of an injured shoulder, and they are sobbing while describing it, it leads me to believe there may be more to the story. It could be an emotional root issue. When you're in this work and do it every day, you learn to feel the vibrations of people. I can tell when someone is emotionally stable just by how their body feels.

I've watched as clients unconsciously rub their leg the whole time they're telling me what is wrong with their shoulder, signaling that the real problem may be with their leg and not necessarily their shoulder. I observed a client recently who was unaware she was flexing her right foot and twisting her right shoulder back while pointing to a pain she felt in her lower back. She came to the clinic because of back pain, but I had a sense that the real issue stemmed from her right ankle. When I worked that ankle, she said, "That's strange! I can feel that in my lower back."

I also pay attention to the words someone uses to describe what's wrong. "I'm a mess" is something we hear a lot when clients walk into our clinic. They use broad strokes and point to "this, that, and the other thing" wrong with them. But once they are on the table, the body will reveal exactly what is going on. The body will never lie. As we work on a person—and it usually doesn't take very many sessions for this to occur—all the red flags will appear. Once we start the moves, the body takes the path of least resistance and starts correcting what it can correct without causing a lot of pain or discomfort. Starting with the first session, the body will get busy correcting each issue and addressing each concern with ease. And then it will get down to the nitty gritty and identify the remaining underlying culprit.

The person will usually come in a few sessions later and state exactly where their root problem is. They will say something like, "Everything else feels great, but there is just one little nagging section right here," and they point somewhere else on their body. What's happened is that the body is organizing more and more in our sessions and making the person's thought process much clearer. Sometimes fixing that last step can cause the body more discomfort for a short amount of time as the body is coming into balance and into organization. I've also seen clarity solidify as quickly as the first session. For example, a new client complains of something and a practitioner is trained to ask, "Why do you feel this way? What caused it? How did you get to this point?" Most clients will have to think about their response—they're not sure. But halfway through the session something will trigger in their brain as the body is coming into organization. All of a sudden, their thoughts become organized and they can recall specific emotional events that likely caused the issue. We don't talk about the specifics of what the event is; we don't need to, because their body already knows how it's going to handle what's surfaced.

Intuitively, I have an idea of what the underlying issue is all along. But I hold back and let the body reveal that issue to the client. I just push the buttons and then allow the body to do what it's supposed to do.

Whatever a client is up against, I find myself assuring them what Mom used to tell me: "This too shall pass." God is a God of order. He did not make our bodies haphazardly. He made human bodies very orderly, so our job in the clinic is to help them stay orderly. When client and practitioner are on the same page and work together to achieve this goal, bodies run like well-oiled machines. And a well-oiled machine doesn't need a mechanic. A tune-up? Yes. As we age, that's exactly what bodywork should be—maintenance on a classic car just to keep it running.

I spent time training my dog, Scout, in the clinic setting because I wanted to explore the role of intuition with animals—and because I love my dog. We would let the clients know we had a dog in the clinic on the days Scout joined me.

One day a man came in with an injury to his ankle—he had slipped on some stairs and his ankle was enormous. I thought maybe he had broken it. Before I touched his ankle, I asked him if it was okay if Scout joined our session. He agreed. I asked if he would take off his socks and shoes on both feet and we'd see which one Scout went to first. It was obvious to me which one was injured, but I didn't know if it would be obvious for a dog. Scout went right to the injured ankle and started licking it. (I had to teach her not to lick!)

Another client agreed to let Scout join her session, and the woman began telling me about some pain her back. Scout sat down before her, looking at her quizzically as she talked. Then Scout got up and went to both of her wrists and sniffed each one. The lady was taken aback and said, "Well, that's strange. I wasn't even going to tell you about the issues with my wrists because I figured you couldn't do anything with those." Thanks, Scout!

When Scout grew tired, she padded her way up to the front reception area to sit with my former receptionist, Suzanne. Scout positioned herself so that she could see every door down the hall in the clinic, giving her a full view of everything going on. She was off the clock, but still very much tuned in.

From the time I started teaching her commands at 10 weeks of age, Scout has proven extraordinary at picking up skills quickly and easily. Sometimes too easily! One night, an over-the-top client with a big personality came in for her session. She's an intense woman, and I love her to pieces. The client went to the restroom, and I ran into my office to get something. Scout is always on my heels most of the time, so she came with me.

This woman doesn't open a door like the average person does—she whips them open. Which is exactly what she did when she came out of the restroom. Scout was startled and growled, and I told her to calm down. The lady put up her hand and remarked, "Don't you judge me, dog. You don't know me." I started laughing—this is just the way this woman is. But I had seen Scout react this way only one other time, and that was with a man in our neighborhood I often saw meandering outside smoking pot. Scout did not like him. My dog is not aggressive, but I had to hold her down one time because I thought she was going to take him out!

To my surprise, when I tried to enter the treatment room and work on the lady, Scout stubbornly stood in front of the doorway and would not let me go in. I assured her it was okay, since the client didn't mind if Scout came into the room with me. Finally, Scout let me pass. My client was face down on the table when I began working. Scout went directly to her open purse and pulled out a vaping pen. The look on my dog's face was full of pride, and I imagined her thinking, "OMG! Look what I just found! I tried to tell you!"

I was horrified and tried giving Scout a subtle signal,

cutting with my finger across my neck. "No! Stop!" I mouthed so I wouldn't disturb my client.

Scout tilted her head at me, confused and disappointed that I wasn't as impressed by her discovery. When I sharply pointed to the purse for Scout to put it back, she reluctantly returned the vaping pen. For the next few minutes, Scout would look hopefully at me and then cock her eyes over at the purse. Cute, but no.

When I left the client to rest after performing a series of moves, I took Scout out of the room with me. Then I thought of something. I went back inside and asked my client, "Is there any way you were around any illicit drugs in the last 24 hours?"

My client was not upset by this inquiry at all. Recreational use of marijuana is legal in Arizona, and I knew her well enough to ask. "Oh, yes! I have anxiety, so I took a hit out in your parking lot."

I nodded. That explained Scout's alarm. We finished the session, and everyone was happy. Scout used her intuition to assume my client was someone she shouldn't like, simply by way of association with my neighbor.

I learned some other interesting insights by testing the intuition a dog would have in the clinic setting. First, I don't think all dogs have it. They're just like people—some people have it and some people don't. Nevertheless, intuition is a learned skill. I teach it to my practitioners by encouraging them to be quiet and observe everything they can about a human body before them on the table. Potential practitioners must come to the practice of body and nerve restoration with a willingness to learn, a natural curiosity, and some degree of tactile sensitivity. They have to be able to feel the difference between a fine strand of hair from a person's head and a quill from a feather. There's a difference, ever so slight.

Intuition and curiosity go hand in hand. I'm driven to learn and study why the world is the way it is and why people are the way they are. When I was young, I didn't have a lot of free time. But when I did, I was usually outside watching the clouds go by, being fascinated by a bug making its way across the grass or just sitting and wondering about life. They say, "Curiosity killed the cat, but satisfaction brought it back." I'm that cat.

Curiosity led me to want to be an astronaut when I was a teenager. The United States had landed the first humans on the moon in 1969, and NASA captivated the attention of the world with its series of Apollo spaceflight programs. There were many nights on the farm in Michigan when I spent hours daydreaming and gazing up at the stars and planets against the darkened sky above me. What was out there? I had to know.

I thought I was smart enough and physically fit enough from my years of working on the farm to meet the demands of being an astronaut. There was only one thing in my past that I felt could possibly hold me back from making my dreams of traveling in outer space come true. So I kept my back super strong and considered all the ways I could hide the fact that I had broken my spine and spent several months in traction.

Then one day I confided my starlit plans to Mom. "I'm thinking I could become an astronaut," I told her as I helped her prepare dinner for our family. As was her way, Mom could communicate whole sentences just by giving us a look or simply nodding her head.

To my dismay, she just continued stirring a dish on the stove and shook her head "no."

I remained silent.

"You need to keep your feet on the ground, Lynell," she assured me with a small smile.

End of conversation. But it didn't keep me from having a wild sense of wonder.

As an adult, I strive to be content but always retain that curious sense of wonderment. *Why are there stars? And what is their purpose? What is the meaning?* Questions like these drive my husband nuts. We walk our dog in the morning and after dark in the evening so I can see stars. Pete cautions me to watch where I'm stepping because I'm often looking straight up at the night sky. He knows my head is full of questions in those moments. "Why are you asking these questions when you know you'll never find the answers?" he'll sometimes joke, scratching his head at his wife.

Our culture, on the other hand, has a disconnect with nature and almost no curiosity. I wish everyone could grow up on a farm or at least spend a year on a farm during their lifetime. It's so easy to lose our sense of wonder. Observational skills and intuition have been replaced with electronic gadgets that do the work for us. We turn to the Internet if we have a question because it has the supposed answer, forgetting that the answer may just be someone's opinion. Nevermind that it may just be a theory, not a fact. Whatever happened to struggling with questions and using your imagination instead to work out an answer? Whatever happened to challenging ourselves to learn one to three new things every day? At the least, it keeps your brain sharp. (Just learning how to work your iPhone can keep you busy learning new things every day!)

Our sense of wonder has all but disappeared today. It's better to fill our minds with nature and ask questions. Go outside. Look up. Stop anxiety from endlessly rolling around in your head and get it out by moving your body. I go for a run, do yoga, work in my garden, or tackle one of the house projects on my list. I am rarely tired, and I love to work. People who move feel better. People who don't move regularly, when they do start again, experience discomfort so they don't continue. My recommendation is to start with just 15 minutes of some activity you enjoy and stick with it. You may be irritated at first, but eventually you'll be glad you did.

Dad used to tell us to go dig fence post holes whenever we were stressed. The first 15 minutes of digging we spent cursing and mouthing off to him under our breath. The next 15 minutes weren't so bad. At the end of the job, we were usually whistling.

Why is that? We grew calm because our heads were clear of stress. We'd pounded it out through our hands onto a piece of equipment and into the ground. When my daughter went through the typical middle school hormonal stage, I'd sometimes be able to get her out of a bad mood by helping me move rocks outside in our yard. Hard labor outside under a blue sky will clear your thoughts. When I am overloaded or can't figure something out, I work out in my yard, go for a run, or do something intense. Getting outside and sweating has many benefits. It's good for your mind and your body.

When I'm not wondering about stars, I find it endlessly intriguing how and why people get better. Not everyone can effectively pursue this line of work. They need to be sensitive people. Anyone overly logical or too analytical has a difficult time with using intuition and struggles to draw insights about life from their environment. Instead, they prefer to rely on facts over sensory information. However, there must be balance. Practitioners must be sensitive people, but if someone is too emotional and not grounded, they "take it all in," and it's way too much and they're not effective.

It's a human tendency to want to be someone or something you are not. That's especially detrimental for someone wanting a career in body work. When a practitioner attempts to be anything other than a facilitator of the work the body is responsible for doing, they're trying to "fix" the body in their own strength. That's misguided. I always remind people when I lead training that we are *not* there to tell the body what to do. We are there to give it some direction, and then it needs to choose what it wants to do. Most of the time the body will choose to heal. Sometimes not, and we have to respect that.

I struggle with this myself because I have a "fix-it" personality, but I have a greater responsibility to the body I'm working with. Some practitioners try to be the fixers instead of becoming more of a channel for God to "fix" that person.

They are often the ones who falter and burn out in this career. Some practitioners are controlling. It comes across in a nice way, and you'd never see it as being negative. But they take on clients' problems and are frustrated when they can't make it better. Then they blame themselves for not doing a good job. I think of Mom wanting to control everything to an impossible degree. She became ill from doing that, and I've seen more than one practitioner become physically ill from control issues. Then they leave a profession they loved.

That's why I say transference in any kind of therapy is a real thing—but it's less about energy transference between client and practitioner and more about control. If a practitioner takes on all the positive energy from someone, they can't help but take on all the negative too when things don't go as they want them to go. And that's no good. If you are not healthy mentally, physically, emotionally, you will not be much help to anyone else. I tell potential practitioners the truth. It's a lot of money, first of all, to learn body and nerve restoration work. Second, if you're going to do it, why wouldn't you want to do it to the best of your ability?

Again, I'm no exception to this struggle. I can't see what is happening on the inside of the human body. I have to be at peace that someone is improving without always having the privilege of observing why or how that is happening. We may never know in some cases why some people recover, and some don't. And we must be content with the answer, whatever it is. It's a mystery.

At the beginning of Robb's transformation, we were on fast-forward and things were clicking along rapidly. He was over the moon excited. When he got to a plateau the first time, I almost allowed his disappointment to overtake me, which is unusual because I am not a negative person.

One day after a period of little progress, he said, "I think this is as far as we can go."

I told him maybe he was right, and then I caught myself. I regrouped because what I really believed was that this was just a plateau of healing.

"You have to be at this plateau in order for everything else to catch up with the progress you've made," I assured him. That was at least my best guess.

I didn't know how long the healing plateau would last because this was new to me, too. My hunch was that it would last only as long as the body and brain needed it to last. And then we were going to jump to the next level. As I said, healing was taking place the whole time; he was just healing on the inside. The nervous system and all the cells were being knitted together, and that took time. After a while, I did another protocol on him, and then he began having more feeling and more movement. He was able to sit up stronger, and all the momentum started building again. I saw the spark and joy return to his face and eyes.

"The only reason I'm still doing this work is because you're still not off your ass walking," I told him. It was my way of telling him how relieved I was that this experiment wasn't over.

"So much pressure," he said sarcastically.

Robb will walk. He is the reason I'm writing this book. Several people have told me for years that I should write a book, but I never wanted to do it. I never understood the point of doing it. Until now. He's like a living miracle. It is unfolding before my eyes, and it's given me more reasons to tell others about the effectiveness of this work.

Clients sometimes ask after a session, "How do you *do* that?" when we help them with an issue. I wish I knew. I don't know how to explain the entire mystery of the body's work. Sometimes this gift is a little unnerving, but overall it is fascinating. My need for control, answers, and understanding wants to know exactly how and why this works. That's the thing I have to learn to let go. I have no idea where this ability is coming from—other than God.

I think about the founder of Bowen, Tom Bowen. Some people questioned his work, and he would always credit God and say he didn't know how to explain it. Others would outright not believe him, or they would even shun him because he couldn't explain his results in a scientific way. There are some things we just can't explain. We have to say it's the God-effect. Our brains can't comprehend that it's brought about by nature. It's that mysterious sense of wonder in life, and we ought to welcome it instead of being frustrated by it.

It still blows my mind today how Robb and other clients like him are getting better. Every day, I tell my practitioners they're bringing a little bit of light to someone's life. That's our job on this earth: being light to each person we meet. That's why I say it's a calling. Life can get heavy and dull, and we're here to help each other find the light.

Decision-making is a test of your intuition. Whatever the decision is, having a sharper sense of wonder, curiosity, and intuition will help you make a better choice.

If you don't decide, you will never move from the spot you're in—physically, emotionally, or mentally. Then you'll find yourself being overly influenced by others, where they're making the decision and you're just following. When I was in my twenties and unsure what to do with my life, I found out quickly that others are happy to fill that void with suggestions of what they think you should do. I felt boxed in with so many opinions, as if I didn't have a say in my own journey. I didn't like that feeling and figured out just in time that I was in charge of myself. I needed to gather my wits and tell myself what to do, because if I didn't—someone else would.

As a young adult, I taught myself to say, "No, thank you" when someone tried to take advantage of me. I went to the mall kiosks where they try to sell you everything under the sun, from sunglasses to timeshares. Patiently, I would listen to their spiel and then say, "No, thank you" and walk away. I did this over and over until I found my voice. I could stand up for myself without worrying about hurting anyone's feelings.

Today it is easy for me to make decisions and set boundaries. Just ask my husband. I married my grounding wire, but I also married young and had to adjust to living together. The very first time I met my husband, he asked for a piece of gum, and I had a feeling I was going to marry him. When I got to know him, I saw that behind those blue eyes was an extraordinarily intelligent mind. The first hurdle popped up when we were engaged and he stayed out past two in the morning, without telling me where he was. There was a terrible storm that night. After talking to everyone I knew trying to find him, I was at a loss. And then I got angry. I stacked his belongings outside the front door and left my ring on the table when I went to work the next day.

When his dad heard about the incident from Pete, he remarked, "I like her! You better get it together, son." I was juggling several jobs then, including my job at Target. Pete came to my register to apologize. I made him stand in line with all the customers, listened to his apology, and said we'd talk later. "You have to leave now and don't get me fired," I warned him. I forgave him. But I stood up for myself and did not let anyone run over me.

Listen to your intuition about what's right for you—everything about you—your life, your health, etc. And remember to course correct as you go. You can always get back on the path if you take a detour. That is the key to every decision you make—sticking with it and following through. The most important action you can take as a parent, for example, is to follow through with consequences when a child crosses the line. It's that simple. When people understand you follow through on what you say, it may frustrate them, but it builds respect.

"Don't make a decision and then waffle," Mom always said. When Pete and I were newlyweds, I asked him more than once not to leave his clothes on the floor. Poor Pete. One day

I threatened to burn them if he did it again. He did it again, and I followed through and tossed them in the fireplace! We stayed married, but his clothes never stayed on the floor again.

That's extreme, but I hope you don't forget what I'm telling you because of this story! It's *essential* to follow through on what's important to you. If you say you're going to do something, do it. You may change the direction of your decision or go through a little roundabout, but you're still going in the same direction. It's like planting a tree when you make a big decision in life. Branch off with little adjustments, but the main decision remains the trunk of the tree. The hardest part about doing anything is deciding. Once the choice is made, just move forward.

God puts the entire puzzle out there for you. It's totally laid out before you, but he's leaving one little piece for you to make a decision on. Are you going to follow through and put that last piece where it goes? Or are you going to hold onto that piece or hide it somewhere and never see what the full picture of your life's purpose could have been?

In business, there is very little emotion involved in my decision making. With a personal decision, the emotional meter will vary between intuition and logic. For many years, I used to fire people for a living in the corporate world, although I did not like that part of the job. My HR background did, however, teach me to weigh options regarding situations and people and do it quickly. What works for me is to think things through logically, and my gut feeling affirms what is making sense to me. I'll also make a pros and cons list, a habit I've done my whole life. For a tough decision, I'll ask myself a series of questions about a particular course of action. Will it serve me? Is it healthy? Will it be safe? Will it serve others well? I run through all those things in my head quite often when I'm making decisions. And then I rely on my intuition and choose.

I've never seen shoulda, coulda, woulda get a person very far, so I don't do it. I challenge you to practice developing your own intuition. Take a step once you "hear" something—you run across an opportunity, you see a chance, you have an inkling—and go in that direction to see what happens next. The only time you fail is when you stop trying. I don't believe in failure. I do, however, believe in learning curves. As Robb said to me one time, "Each time you come across something new is a reminder that you are still moving forward." You have enough spring in your step to jump over life's hurdles. Just keep learning and trying.

8

following your calling

THE TRIP WAS HARD because it held so many memories. The last time I'd hiked this trail to the top of Angels Landing in Zion National Park was with my best friend, Karen, and our young daughters. We did not know at the time that Karen had a deadly brain tumor. I remember she was walking slower than usual and seemed short of breath. She didn't want to go all the way up to the top of the trail, and I didn't blame her. Walter's Wiggles is the near the end of the climb to reach Angels Landing and is extremely steep with 21 switchbacks. Climbing 250 feet of elevation so quickly would wear out anyone, I told myself.

"That's okay," I told Karen that day. "No big deal."

Even as I spoke these words, I fought off this alarming sense that something was definitely wrong with my friend. I tried not to seem overly concerned.

Months later, cancer would overtake Karen. Her daughter,

Cortney, lived with us while her mom was being treated in the hospital, and she and my daughter have remained close all this time.

In 2021, the three of us—Cortney, Analise, and myself—decided to return to Zion to hike the very same trail her mom was unable to complete. When we set out, I was in front and Analise made sure to follow last, hemming in her friend between the two of us like a hen and her chick. We knew deep down that Cortney might have a hard time that day, thinking of her mom and reliving old memories. I was lost in my own thoughts as well when suddenly I didn't sense the girls hiking behind me anymore. I turned to see that Cortney had stopped. She felt as if she couldn't breathe, so we pulled off to the side of the steep trail and waved people forward to pass us. I assured Cortney that we were not in a race and told her to take her time. I worked on her right there on the trail just to get her breathing again and let her breath come through in slow, deep draws.

After a while, Cortney wanted to continue, and I ended up letting the two girls go ahead alone while I went on a different trail. It was a good, healing trip for all of us.

I share this story because not every story has a happy ending like Robb's or like many of the other clients we have the privilege of working with every day. Life comes with challenges and sadness for all of us, and we must make the best of it and not grow discouraged when things don't turn out the way we desperately want them to. We can learn to be okay with God's greater purpose when tragedy occurs.

In fact, the body has its own unique way of dealing with

tragedy and grief. I had a client whose husband had killed himself two years prior, but I didn't know that was part of her story when we first met. She came to the clinic because she felt numb in her arms. I started her face down on the table like I do with most clients, and everything was going well. I left for a rest period to let the moves "simmer," but when I came back in the room to turn her over, she was sobbing.

I gave her some tissues and made a point not to ask her what was wrong. "Let it all out," I encouraged her and left the room again. I peeked in on her a few minutes later and saw she was still crying. So I shut the door and let her continue.

After 20 minutes I went back in and saw she had stopped crying. "I don't think I have cried so hard—ever," she remarked, her eyes red and puffy from fresh tears. Then she shared the story about her husband killing himself. Afterwards, she made an interesting comment. "I feel like I can breathe now," she told me. The numbness in her arms dramatically healed after that day, and she returned to normal function. Now I see her about once every six months, just for a tune up.

Another client, whose child died unexpectedly, developed a strange aversion to swallowing normally and could never take a deep, cleansing breath. She could not swallow a pill and found herself feeling as if she were choking quite often. The client described something being "stuck" in her throat, which I silently related to the grief she felt over her loss. After working with us in our clinic, she processed her grief and regained her ability to swallow normally and take deep breaths.

If you know the story of Genesis in the Bible, it says that God breathed life into Adam. That breath of God is a good picture of what sustains us today. When we're stressed, or sad, or overwhelmed, we're like this grieving client or Cortney on the trail. Life is sometimes so hard that we feel we can't breathe.

Stress, as I've said, leads to shallow breathing, which leads to other problems. We're giving people some air—literally and figuratively—every day in our clinic and giving them some room to breathe. It makes all the difference. I often incorporate taking deep breaths with my clients, and I also take my own advice. One of the reasons why I run is to force myself to breathe deep and pull in as much oxygen as possible. Working hard outside like my father encouraged us to do on the farm accomplishes something similar—pushing yourself to breathe deep as you work helps clear your mind so you can think again and continue another day.

One of Robb's exercises is to sit upright in a chair and take a deep breath through his nose, raising his arms out to the side and above his head. He holds the breath a few seconds before exhaling through his mouth and bringing his arms down at the same time. This exercise pulls in more needed oxygen. When he was developing core strength in his previously paralyzed abdomen and lower torso, I prompted him to keep moving forward in the chair each week, making it a bit more challenging for him to maintain his balance. Today he sits on the edge of a chair and performs this exercise lovely and with perfect control. This routine is helping his body, brain, balance, and breath work together.

The body is capable of healing when it is given a safe space and the right direction. I still don't understand everything about how this works, and if you're scratching your head, just know that I am too. I do know that when the body feels safe, and we gently guide it into order, it will self-correct everything that it can possibly correct.

The hardest part of our job is knowing when *not* to do too much work. It's not good to overload the body with information, forcing it to do a lot of work in a short amount of time. It's overwhelming. Our job is to trust the work—to do a little and trust that the body will do its thing. That is a challenge because naturally we want to do everything possible at once to address a problem. Instead, the goal is to start the process and let the body organize itself.

I'll never forget working on a four-month-old baby girl for the first time. Babies are like electrical panels—push the right buttons and they'll usually be fine. In this case, the mom brought the baby to see us at the clinic because her daughter wouldn't eat very well and was uncomfortable whenever she went down for a nap. She preferred to be propped upright all the time. When I saw the baby, the child's face was red and puffed up as if it were swollen.

I asked if the baby had been taken to a pediatrician, and the mom said yes. The doctors had assured her that it was colic and that the baby would be fine in time. "But there's something really wrong," the mom concluded. "So I was hoping you could figure it out."

I was observing the baby while her mom was talking. I needed to do a specific move in the neck area, but I knew the baby was likely to cry out when I did so.

Her three-year-old sister was with them, so I asked her to

assist us. "Can you stand to the side of your sister and get her to look over at you?" I asked.

The little girl moved to the left side, and the baby tried following her with her eyes. That's when I noticed that the baby could not move her head in that direction at all and seemed short of breath. When the baby tried to look to the left, her face became redder and bigger. I wasn't sure what was wrong, but one thing I did know is that this was *not* just colic. Something was keeping her from moving her head and blocking the air supply. I knew the baby's nervous system was still developing because she was so young, but I was also certain it would be able to take care of the issue restricting the air supply if I targeted the right nerve plexus.

I explained to the mother that I was going to do a few moves on her baby that would make the child uncomfortable but would not cause her pain in any way. "She is going to scream for a split-second only because of the odd sensation that's being produced. Then it will be over, and she'll be better," I said, instructing the mom to sit and hold the baby on her lap.

I asked the big sister to hold the baby's hand and remain on the left side of her. Then I performed four moves around the baby's neck and skull, and we waited for what was probably only 20 seconds but seemed like 20 minutes.

What happened next was startling and assuring at the same time. The baby's head started wobbling, and she screamed once. Then she threw her head back and then forward. As her head came forward, the child took a big gulp of air like she was coming up out of deep water. The baby took in such a big, deep breath that her mom and I wondered aloud when it was going to stop. Suddenly, the baby let out her breath and gave a big smile. Then she began babbling happily, turning her head and looking straight over at her older sister on the left.

The mom burst into tears before she too started laughing with joy. Later, she explained that the baby had been born with the umbilical cord wrapped around her neck. I assumed something like that had happened because of the rigidity of the child's neck and her shallow breath. The nerve plexus was what needed to be targeted to make the correction.

Once the baby was breathing normally, she looked completely different. By the time the family left the clinic, her head did not appear swollen, and her face had returned to a normal flesh color. Even the receptionist noted the remarkable change and commented that she didn't look like the same child.

I work on children, ages birth to nine years of age, at no charge. Each case is as challenging as it is interesting. Another mom brought her baby to the clinic because the child still wasn't walking at 15 months of age. When her mom stood and held the child around her chest in front of her, the baby lifted and held her legs out front instead of releasing them down in a natural walking or standing position. The baby was completely uninterested in trying to walk. Every time the mom tried to put her down on the floor, the baby would just sit in a heap.

While a neurologist might have been an option in a traditional setting, the mom brought the baby to the clinic first to see what we could do to help. After observing and listening to the mom describe the baby's symptoms, I decided to do six moves that I knew would bring results. Again, I also knew it would be temporarily uncomfortable for the baby because her nerves were bundled up inside her hip sockets.

"The moves I perform are going to feel uncomfortable like electric jolts to her, but it will not hurt her," I cautioned her mom.

The child watched with huge brown eyes when I began working. I started with a small rolling move around her low back and into her hip flexors. She screamed a little, as predicted, but then she dropped her legs straight out. The mom was still holding her baby, arms around her chest, and the child's legs dangled straight down in front of her. That was a first. The little girl looked surprised! She took a deep breath and looked over her shoulder at her mother for assurance.

I completed the other moves, but the child did not cry out. She winced once, and then her facial expression became one of relief as she reached to put her feet on the floor. Holding her mom's fingers, she even took a few tentative steps. The mom sent us video a few days later of the baby smiling and walking back and forth between her mom and dad, unassisted, with her arms wide open ready for a hug. The difference was dramatic.

I'm no miracle worker, but I get to see them happen quite often in the clinic. When I think about what I want more of in the next few years, I know for certain that I want more miracles. I expect them—and why not? We see them daily in the clinic. Another one of my goals in the coming years is to teach those who sincerely want to help others how to bring forth those same miracles. I want to train others to learn this work because it's important, and it works.

In the meanwhile, I'm the cleaning crew, the HR person, the chief decision-maker, and a busy practitioner doing what I love. I'm still very much a farmgirl at heart, doing my chores and cleaning the building with my husband each week. You know, staying busy morning to night. I felt at home when one of my clients named Heather invited me to her horse ranch. I am not necessarily a horse fan because those big guys scare me. But my daughter wanted to learn how to ride, so my client and I traded services. I experimented with some bodywork on her horses in exchange for horse lessons for Analise.

A giant horse named Mia was so tall I had to use a stepstool to reach her back. The first time I worked on Mia, she laid down and went to sleep immediately! My client tied Mia's halter to the gate the next time so she wouldn't lie down on me while I was trying to work. The same thing also happened one time when I flew to Michigan to visit Dad on the farm. I asked him if I could work on one of his cows that was sickly. He didn't know what was wrong, and I did not either. But I wanted to see if I could help. Dad held the cow next to the fence as I worked, and in the process the 1500-pound animal fell completely asleep.

"I don't know what you're doing, but it works," Dad said later, explaining that the cow slept for many hours after I worked on it and it recuperated the next day.

One day after I had been working on a horse named Socks for several days at Heather's ranch, I drove up to the barn and had just stepped out of my car when Socks charged out of the barn and bee lined toward me.

"Don't move!" Heather called, running after Socks in her boots.

Backing up against the side of my car, I tried to look small and stand still. The horse screeched to a halt in front of me, then reached his head around my shoulder, and gently pulled me to him. He let out a satisfied snort as he held me in this horse-hug, and I warmed up to the idea as I slowly patted his neck lightly.

Heather was laughing when she reached my car. The animal had been troubled with hip pain for some time, she explained, and my work had helped give him some relief. This was his way of telling me thank you, she assured me. Those days at the ranch made me even more appreciative that humans can explain exactly where they hurt and provide feedback, although getting a horse hug is not so bad!

Information is power when it relates to your health. But can it be too much information? Yes, especially if you are looking in the wrong direction for help. If you're just sitting in front of the boob tube absorbing all that the commercials are telling you about symptoms that you may or may not have (but now you're convinced that you *do* have), you're exposing yourself to rhetoric, not helpful information.

People often ask me what simple actions they could take to start living life as we're meant to live it—and immediately see a change in their health. I'll start with touch. As I've said, practitioners feel energy and vibration. We move our hands around the whole body to see what is going on because the power of touch is imperative to our work. If people aren't touched in a caring and safe way, they are apt to grow cold, as if they don't know how to respond to touch or to people. Studies have proven that if a baby is not lovingly touched, he or she won't thrive. If you touch a baby gently, even to soothe a bellyache, they calm down, they're soothed, and then they heal. Skin is the largest organ in the body, and it's designed to protect you. Anything that is alive needs to be touched. Even animals love touch. Our 80-pound dog loves it when our five-pound cat cleans her face and ears. Scout will paw lightly at the cat, rolling over onto her back to be more accessible.

I believe "caring touch" awakens the following: creativity, the senses, healing and repair, direction (when needed), and clarity of the mind and heart. The Creation account in Genesis tells us that God made us with his hands. Touch is that imperative to human beings and brings us back to some sort of creation or creativity inside each of us. It also awakens and sharpens all our senses if we're touched lovingly.

Touch also awakens healing because of the type of work we do. When I'm working on a client, they often say they feel the electrical buzz I've described in earlier chapters. That's my signal to point out their body is practicing good communication. "Your body is alive inside," I tell them.

Others may register a touch and say something like, "It's tapping over here now" and they point to their shoulder or hip. I tell them the hammers are "tapping things back into order." It's just a visual to help people understand the sensations. You don't feel your skin on a regular basis; you know you have it, but you don't feel it. You just go about your day—until something happens to that skin and then you pay attention to it.

Touch seems to awaken repair; it awakens whatever is dormant in the body, either to heal, or create new pathways and connections, or grow, or to soothe. Touch also provides clarity and direction, when needed. We've all experienced how a soothing touch can comfort someone who is hurting. Relieving stress for someone can help clear their mind so they can make good decisions about their life.

When a client gets up off the table after a session and says, "I've never felt anything like this before," I'm reminded of the incredible power of touch. They say things like, "I felt like I was floating," or, "I was seeing colors—how is that possible?" I just smile. These remarkable observations are not all that remarkable; they're just normal healthy body processes. Synapses are firing and doing their everyday work. We tend to think it's something extraordinary because it's been so long since they did their job properly without being hindered.

The body doesn't need complication in the healing process. It is already complicated enough. The body requires very simplistic encouragement on different levels. In Robb's case, for example, I didn't want him taking any supplements for the first three years we worked together. I wanted to see what his body was capable of with the most pure and simplistic messages.

Once I started to see muscle tissue thriving and rebuilding and signals reconnecting, that marked the time to support and encourage this progress using supplements. Supplements helped his body repair nerve sheathing, so the messages traveled a little smoother and easier. His body doesn't have to work so hard now that things are rebuilding. Before, however, supplements would have been too much, too soon. He didn't have enough signaling or muscle tissue for the body to make use of supplementation. Had I supplemented too early in the process, all it would do is give him a stomachache since there was not enough muscle tissue to absorb it. Modern advertising says your body is incapable of healing without the help of a certain pill, but I like to see what the body is capable of on its own *before* supplementation or medicine. And then if we need to supplement, we will supplement, but my strategy is to do that gently, not just throw pills at symptoms.

Here is another example. A client in her seventies had her liver enzymes tested at the doctor, and they were off the charts. "But I'm not a drinker or smoker," she said, perplexed at these readings.

I asked if she was taking anything.

"Only supplements, all natural," she replied.

I asked her how she knew what supplements to take, and she said she was following suggestions from her friend.

"Is your friend a naturopath, or a nutritionist, or a doctor?" I inquired. I have a good rapport with this client, as we have worked together many years, so she knew where I was going.

"Well, no..." she answered slowly.

I've learned to take age out of the equation when determining what someone should or should not know by now. I asked her to tell me all the supplements she was taking.

When she mentioned she was taking Kava Kava root, I stopped her. Why was she taking that?

"It's for stress," came the reply.

"Yes, but why are *you* taking it?" She said that she had been very stressed out lately, and her friend told her to take it.

When I asked what, if anything, she knew about this supplement. My client smiled sheepishly and said, "Only what was on the box…"

I took one of my holistic medicine books from college off the shelf and asked her to read a paragraph aloud. She then read how Kava Kava is one of several supplements that needs to be taken with great caution. It can be detrimental to the liver if not taken under supervision and can even damage the liver in short order.

"Oh my gosh! What should I do?" she cried.

I advised that she stop taking it. "What we're doing today will help your body de-stress naturally," I added. Then I will give you other things to do like breathing exercises—simple things that will not harm you. Have your doctor check your liver enzymes in three months, and it should be right back to normal."

And it was.

Clients are often too trusting of "all natural" herbs and tinctures and disregard caution when taking them. The problem is that these are much more potent because they are closer to the source. We have to educate ourselves on whatever we put in our body—even if it's all natural, it may not be right for you.

Another male client's blood pressure readings were all

over the place. No one knew why. Maybe it was the fact that his cholesterol was also high that the doctors wanted to put him on a series of statin drugs to lower his cholesterol. When he came to see me, I suggested drinking lemon water every morning and eating a cup of fresh pineapple every day, since pineapple and other foods are known to break down plaque. His blood pressure went down after a series of six sessions, and it has maintained a normal level. I was blessed with common sense from both my parents, and like my parents taught me long ago, food is your friend.

A client in his early fifties was diagnosed with high pressure behind his eyes. His eye pressure measured 30 and 32 at the eye doctor. I asked him to pop by six times over a matter of weeks to focus on his eye nerves, cervical plexus, and Vagus nerve. Then he had his eyes rechecked at the doctor, and the pressures had dropped to 18 and 19. The look on his face was priceless. Again, what we do at the clinic doesn't follow a traditional approach, but it works.

Another client in her seventies was diagnosed with osteoporosis after her bone density test. Her doctor wanted her to start taking medicine immediately to correct the issue. She came to our clinic because she didn't want to take medicine because of the potential side effects and wondered if there was something else she could do to strengthen her bones. I suggested she begin regular weight training, starting with two-pound weights or soup cans.

"Oh, that won't work. It's too late—I'm too old," she said.

She is an avid golfer but had never lifted weights in her life. It's not too late, I explained. I also suggested she start and end her day with five jumping jacks. Low-impact exercise encourages the body to lay down more bone. Once she began doing the low-impact exercises and lifting weights, increasing the weight as she progressed, she developed more muscle and bone mass. Her next bone density test revealed the positive results.

"Look! I have muscle here! And here!" she said the next time I saw her, proudly pointing to her legs and arms. It takes effort to take care of ourselves—it doesn't happen automatically.

Some influential leaders in the fields of science and technology want to mesh Artificial Intelligence with humans in the name of improving our lives. I saw an interview many years ago with a prominent leader in technology and have not forgotten it. In my opinion, that's not where we should be going into the future. We need to go back to origination, as Tom Bowen often emphasized. We need to go back to tilling dirt and farming. Farming today has been taken over by huge companies and industrialized. That's why Dad got out of it after Mom died. He said he couldn't compete with the big boys. Relying on a faceless, industrial-driven world for our food or living in a virtual world where nothing is real is not appealing to me. I want life to be real for myself and my family, and I want that for others.

Exercise is also at the top on my list for maintaining good health. At least get out and walk. I'm adamant that you must get outside, not always doing your exercise in the house or in a gym. The fresh air will do you wonders.

Next, get off the phones and computers. Shut them down.

Phones are not allowed in my clinic, and I've been known to confiscate if need be.

Enjoy a dinner plate of colorful food every night. Eat and enjoy all things in moderation. Nothing should be over the top, no matter what it is. Nothing extreme on any front. "Eat and drink everything real, in moderation, and you will be just fine," as my great-grandmother used to say. In her generation, nothing in her kitchen came out of a cardboard box. When you go in a store today, stay out of the middle aisles of processed foods, and shop only the fresh fruits, veggies, meat, and dairy on the outside aisles.

Soul care is another way to take the best care of your physical body. If you fill your cup with fear, anxiety, and anger, you will become bitter and unhealthy. Bitter people often tend to have more health issues, including dangerous consequences from habitually overeating to soothe their anxiety and bitterness. Did you know that deep anger and resentment can also show up as arthritis in the body? Anyone can have arthritis, but it's not a coincidence that I often see it paired with deep, angry, bitter emotions that haven't been dealt with in a healthy way.

Physical pain may be related to an emotional issue. It can be tied to their low back where the body's emotional state is seated. Or, as I explained in an earlier chapter, it could be something in their gut causing the concern since the gut houses the powerful enteric nervous system—the second brain. Sometimes the body is so overwhelmed that it can't issue a direct message and pinpoint exactly what's wrong. In a panic, the body begins throwing any red flags it can to get help, and we must weed through those flags to find the main issue.

I've seen so many examples of emotional pain points in the body. Clients will come in with swollen or locked up knees and tell me they "didn't do anything" to cause it. If you listen to their stories, however, the pain often has to do with a relationship they need to deal with in their inner circle. It doesn't have to be a spouse—just someone within their circle of friends or family. Your hips can ache if you can't seem to make a good decision about moving forward. Sometimes you're stuck, trying to make a decision. Or you're not happy about a decision. Or sometimes you're just hesitant about the decision—and suddenly your hip may start aching out of the blue. When I hear stories that connect hip pain with decision-making, I want to say, "If you make the wrong decision and fail, pick yourself up and try it again."

I am a three-tries person. I always have been. If you try something three times and it fails three times, then you need to change direction. Do it quickly and don't waste time. The circumstances will tell you which direction you're supposed to go. I live by that three-tries rule. With any big decision I need to make, if I hear an affirmation in a certain direction three times, good or bad, then I know which way I will go. I always, always get three affirmations. My former receptionist and friend, Suzanne, even keeps count for me! I lean heavily on that principle whenever I face a fork in the road. I'll blast my husband or a close friend with my thoughts and options. Then I'll think and pray about it, and I won't move on anything until I've received three indications of what the right choice is.

Another emotional pain point is ankle pain. And it is often tied to neglecting tedious to-dos that you know you need to do but you don't want to do them. There are lists of emotional connections with each joint in the body. The point is to realize the complexity of your body and trust what it's trying to tell you about what parts of your life need attention.

None of the above suggestions about physical and emotional health cost money. It's so simple, but it's hard for people to be uncomplicated with their health matters because they often overthink it. I lead by example in all these areas. I don't suggest anything I haven't first tried myself.

When I stop to look around at how far we've come as a company, I remember the days at one of my smaller offices where two full chairs meant standing room only. There was just enough heat in the place for the lobby and one treatment room. By that time, I'd made inroads and connections in the community of Prescott. Many firefighters at a station down the road would whoop and holler as they drove by, just to say hi. The street was also popular with the Harley crowd, who rumbled into town and unknowingly disturbed my clients' restful bliss.

After working in two small offices, I moved our growing business to another building we called The Bunker. Plywood lined the walls of the clinic, and one wall was actually a cleverly disguised garage door. We regularly escorted rogue lizards out using a waste basket and a manilla file folder cover. Denise had hand warmers in her pockets, and she wore her parka while charting. I brought the dirty laundry home every night.

When we moved to yet another building and had room for five chairs in the waiting room, hot water in the bathroom, an on-site laundry, and a file room, I thought I was in heaven. The office offered lots of sunshine, ample parking, and a training room upstairs. What more could we want? But we continued to grow, so in the fall of 2017, we moved into our largest facility (with real walls) and are still there today at Lynell & Company, a Body and Nerve Restoration Center.

One of my best decisions in business was to not be afraid of success. Deep down, many people are a little afraid of the increased exposure and responsibility that come with it. Once you start making a name for yourself or your business, you may run into self-doubt. When I started out, I just wanted to stay in my corner and didn't want many people to know who I was. I hesitated until I became convinced that I had to trust myself regardless of what others thought.

After I officially changed the name of the business to Lynell & Company in 2012, I had heart palpitations when I saw my name going up on a big sign out front. But I asked myself, "Do you want to be successful, or don't you? Make up your mind." I had to lose my fear of being successful and let go of the part of me that wanted to remain anonymous. I'm often told that my company has the largest quantity of clients in this field in the United States, and I've personally worked on over 10,000 bodies in my tenure. We remain booked solid throughout the year, year after year. If you can trust and believe in yourself, then you ought to welcome success and remember that other people's opinions of what you do have no bearing.

There is no way I could do what we are doing alone. I love employing good people and watching them do their work, happy and fulfilled. That's my HR experience coming out in me, but I do enjoy seeing what people are made of. I like surprising them with the realization that they can do some amazing things to help others. It is so satisfying to me when people who work with me believe in themselves.

I also love being part of a community like Prescott that has been so willing to help us grow as a company. When you feel at home among people who have given you so much, you want to give back. Our clinic donates a few days a year to help groups in our community, like the military, by offering free body and nerve sessions to anyone who needs it. We start in the morning and finish late at night to accommodate those who come to see us. Every other spring, I also invite my sister Donna, who is a nurse, to host a talk about breast health at our clinic. Our company also participates in an annual food drive. Instead of paying for a session, clients bring a bag of food to donate to the food bank. One year we donated several carloads packed with food. The food bank was facing a shortage that day, with a line of people growing outside on the sidewalk. Their staff and our staff started crying as we realized the timing of our unannounced visit that day was perfect.

In the future, I would like to focus on training, including a certification process for practitioners and continuing education hours for credit. So many practitioners are already doing the work beautifully, but they have the potential to improve and create even better results with training. The way I train practitioners is the same way my mother taught me to make a pie crust in the kitchen of our home in Michigan. She taught me to make the ruffle around the edge of the crust with my thumb and forefinger, standing side-by-side as I worked my pie, and showing me each step with her own pie. I usually completed a handful of ruffles by the time hers was in the oven! Likewise, I show my practitioners a move, then they repeat it as we stand side-by-side. The body gives us the feedback we need. The difference between our execution of the moves is the same as the difference between Mom and me—experience.

I would like to explore having the top practitioners who serve with us to open branches of our Body and Nerve Restoration Center around the country. A practitioner in the Northwest, for example, is a former masseuse who asked me to train her. She doubled, tripled, and then quadrupled her business in one year. I'm also developing other referrals in other states to reach even more people using qualified practitioners I've trained. It's a lot of hours and it's intense, but the practitioners get their hands on so many bodies, which solidifies what they're learning, body after body.

I also envision developing a grant program for special clients like Robb so practitioners can donate their time to help with the extended care they need. I think clients like him have already had so much taken from them. I believe you must have a calling and a true desire to help others in this business and not make it about the almighty dollar. The health care profession faces the same temptation all companies face—to cut corners because of the potential of fast, easy money. That has nothing to do with a calling. I've seen the love of money ruin those in this line of work who take advantage of others.

What we do in my clinic is hard work and requires serious training. I believe you must be willing to work hard in this field. I do not allow "woo woo" and hocus pocus to come in and take over in my clinic. And I don't do weird. Our work is not woo woo, and it's not easy. That's one of the highest compliments a client can give when they say, "This isn't weird at all!" I don't know if they're looking for crystals and magic tricks, but the way I run my clinic goes back to my appreciation for common sense and how logical the body is. The world has enough weird in it, don't you think?

This is the story of how I found my calling. But what about yours? I believe everyone has a calling in life. But it's possible for people to miss it. It's tempting for our ego to get in our own way. We are easily persuaded to do what we want to do...or think we *should* do. Instead, try carving out more time to be quiet and intuitive enough to see that maybe you're being pointed in another direction. People who can set aside what *they* think they want to do with their time on this earth will usually stumble onto something bigger and better that they're meant to do.

I'm a big believer of having God in your life. If someone doesn't have a sure foundation in life, they are like a leaf blowing in the wind with no idea what they're grabbing onto, or where they're going to land next. Try listening more and being quiet and see if you don't hear the next clue about what you're supposed to do with the time we're all given.

People who don't know my story often say how lucky I am to have found my purpose. But those who know me well, including you if you've made it this far in the book, also know that I had no clue what I was doing for so long. My path to what I do now was not a straight line. That would have been too boring. Before I found this work, I was going through the motions every day, convinced there had to be more to life, but not sure what it was. Now I know for sure that life is more than just the daily grind. There *has* to be more than we're born, we live, we die. That's not logical, and God is very logical. There is some kind of smokescreen obscuring what's really there, and I plan to figure it out one day at a time.

Although this is my story, maybe you can see yourself or your friend within these pages. I watched how Dad used his hands for good in so many ways throughout my life. Even though it took me a while to see how he passed on his compassion to me, I'm thankful I was given the opportunity and the wisdom to grasp onto his gift. Using my hands as a vessel of healing for others has filled my cup with great compassionate rewards.

For so long I didn't know my purpose. So I tuned in to my environment, and all the people and circumstances in it, trying to figure it out. I am a very good listener, so I strung together my desire to learn new things with what I heard Mom say about having my father's hands. I paid attention when Klaus gave me the bodywork instructor's business card. Because I listened and heard something that interested me, I listened a little more and took a step in that direction just to see where it led me. I was persistent enough to keep asking the instructor to teach me and didn't give up when she said no at first. And thank God I was brave enough to show up at that first class without having any prior experience.

I have no idea exactly what is next for me, but I feel as if I'm halfway there. I developed that strong sense after four years of seeing Robb improve so drastically, especially during the most recent months of his therapy. One of my goals in writing this book was to capture a few of the insights I've learned about the human body and healing because I sense my future will be spent educating and training others to continue learning and growing in this work long after I'm gone. Another goal was to share how I found my life's purpose. It started with my father's hands and led me to a place where I can use my hands to guide others to hope and healing. Still, I don't feel that I have reached my destiny yet. I tend to think that my calling is the road to my destiny, and I'm sure I'll get there one day. In the meantime, I'm going to stay on that road until I get there. How about you?

When our calling is the path that we are already on, life moves us along from point to point. We move, we change jobs, etc. As we arrive at each new station in life, our challenge is to learn all we can there and grow until we reach the next station. It's like Robb pounding it out on the treadmill. When he hits the next phase of healing and the next, he is that much more enthusiastic and committed to doing all he can to reach his ultimate goal of walking again. It's like Scout and I on one of our runs through the woods—when we sense we're making progress and we're almost home, the two of us pick up the pace because we're excited to reach the end.

We're all running a great race on the way to our final destination. May I remind you to take time to look up, and not stare at your shoes? Look around at the wonder and mystery of life happening all around you every day. Stay curious. Ask questions. Get outside more and take a deep, cleansing breath of good, fresh air. Your body is way more capable than we give it credit for. Take care of it on your own journey of health and healing, and you'll find you're getting stronger and wiser with every mile. Just promise me you won't stop running until you reach the end.